P9-CPV-431

The Art of
NURSING

About the Cover

Bamboo and Rocks

Bamboo, pine, and plum blossoms are prized as the "three friends of winter."
For Li K'an (1245–1320), the artist who painted these shoots and branches, the study
and painting of bamboo was a special calling. In his *Bamboo Treatise* he wrote:

> When bamboo starts to grow, it is only a tender sprout of about an inch, yet all
> the joints and leaves are there. From the tiny size of a cicada chrysalis and the scale of
> a snake's skin to that of giant blades of a hundred feet, a bamboo is born complete with
> all its parts. Yet some bamboo painters draw a single joint at a time, and pile up leaves
> one by one; this way how can they capture the bamboo? To paint bamboo one must
> have the complete bamboo in one's breast. Holding a brush and carefully surveying the
> silk, the painter sees what he wants, then quickly moves the brush to catch what he
> sees. It is like going after a hare or a falcon; if there is the slightest hesitation, the
> opportunity is gone.

From *Spring Flowers Autumn Moons: The Flowers and Gardens of Ancient China.* The
Metropolitan Museum of Art, 1984.

Cover art: The Metropolitan Museum of Art, Gift of the Dillon Fund, 1973. (1973.120.7ab)
Photograph © 1983 The Metropolitan Museum of Art.

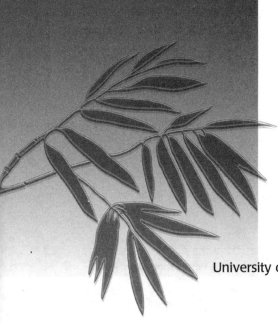

Carolyn Cooper, PhD, RN
Clinical Associate Professor
School of Nursing
University of North Carolina at Chapel Hill
Chapel Hill, North Carolina

The Art of
NURSING

....

A PRACTICAL INTRODUCTION

Saunders

An Imprint of Elsevier

SAUNDERS
An Imprint of Elsevier
The Curtis Center
Independence Square West
Philadelphia, PA 19106

Library of Congress Cataloging-in-Publication Data

Cooper, Carolyn, RN.
    The art of nursing : a practical introduction / Carolyn Cooper.
        p. ; cm.
    Includes bibliographical references.

    ISBN-13: 978-0-7216-8216-7   ISBN-10: 0-7216-8216-2
    1. Nursing. 2. Nurse and patient. I. Title.
    [DNLM: 1. Nursing Care—methods. 2. Knowledge. 3. Nurse-Patient Relations.
WY 100 C776a 2001]
    RT41.C7787 2001
    610.73—dc21

                         00-033000

Cover art: The Metropolitan Museum of Art, Gift of the Dillon Fund, 1973. (1973.120.7ab)
Photograph © 1983 The Metropolitan Museum of Art.

THE ART OF NURSING: A PRACTICAL INTRODUCTION

ISBN-13: 978-0-7216-8216-7
ISBN-10: 0-7216-8216-2

Copyright © 2001 by Saunders

All rights reserved. No part of this publication may be reproduced or transmitted in any form
or by any means, electronic or mechanical, including photocopy, recording, or any information storage and retrieval system, without permission in writing from the publisher.

Permissions may be sought directly from Elsevier's Health Sciences Rights
Department in Philadelphia, PA, USA: phone: (+1) 215 239 3804, fax: (+1) 215 239 3805,
e-mail: healthpermissions@elsevier.com. You may also complete your request on-line
via the Elsevier homepage (http://www.elsevier.com), by selecting 'Customer Support'
and then 'Obtaining Permissions'.

Printed in the United States of America

Last digit is the print number: 9   8   7

In memory of my parents
Owen Cooper and Elizabeth Thompson Cooper

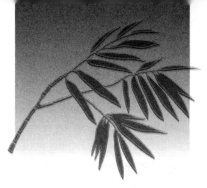

Preface

··

The idea for this book grew out of the need for a nursing text that focused on the art of nursing. For several years I have taught an introduction to nursing course. I have relied on a wide variety of sources including the stories of nurses, fiction, and poetry to help students envision the diversity and richness embodied in the artful practice of nursing. In formal evaluations of the course, students overwhelmingly report that a favorite aspect of the course is the stories about nursing. Further, graduates of the program regularly cite "the stories" as the outstanding memory from this first nursing course.

This text, which features the stories of expert nurses as they portray artful nursing practice, was inspired in large part by my students' enthusiasm for the lasting quality and power of good nursing stories. The usefulness of reading and discussing nurse narratives resides in the student's capacity for developing an appreciation for the nuances of the expert nurse's response. As students recognize in nurse stories the fine distinctions of artful nursing practice, they begin to envision how their own repertoire of responses could be attuned to the stories of individual patients. This occurs because aspects of the narratives remain in the heart and the mind's eye after the story has been read.

This text has two sections. The first three chapters describe the knowledge nurses use and how they attain that knowledge. In the second section the focus is on seven concepts central to the art of nursing. The actualization of artful nursing is as broad and creative as the nurse's imagination and skill; hence this depiction of the art of nursing is far from complete. Further, no attempt has been made to join the developing commentary in the nursing literature about the nature or scope of the art of nursing. Rather the concepts depicted in this text represent some of the common themes in artful nursing practice. Specific concepts were selected based upon the substance of each nurse's story and the usefulness of supporting nursing literature.

Each chapter begins with an introduction of the highlighted concept designed to acquaint students with key aspects of the concept. The nurse narrative that constitutes the heart of each chapter follow this. A discussion and analysis of the concept as it was actualized in the narrative and a description of challenges to the enactment of the concept are also included. Group and individual exercises designed to help students explore the application of the concept to their own developing understanding of nursing practice conclude each chapter.

Ten individuals were interviewed for this text. In some cases the individual nurse's story is largely unaltered; in other cases aspects of several stories have been combined to fully depict the concept. However, every part of the stories in this text is true, representing what has actually taken place and what continues to occur in diverse forms on countless occasions in the private encounters between nurses and their patients.

Students are encouraged to imagine themselves as the nurse as they read these stories and to pay attention to the feelings that arise. Notice the facts, but also notice what it feels like to be an expert nurse. The Application section of each chapter will help the student identify his or her own responses to the nurse's actions.

I owe much to co-workers whose generosity enabled this endeavor. Colleagues Sandy Funk and Elizabeth Tornquist initially challenged me to write. My dean, Cindy Freund, awarded me a Carrington leave, freeing me to write unencumbered for a semester. Other faculty served as informal consultants, including Carol Durham, Yvonne Eaves, Beverly Foster, Rosalie Hammond, Jane Kaufman, Maureen Kelley, Diane Kjervik, Barbara Germino, Chris McQuiston, Judy Miller, Mary Ann Peter, Rachel Stevens, and Betty Woodard.

Friends and family who have encouraged me in this process include Helen Ashby, Edith Back, Jean Blackwell, Elizabeth Cooper, Ruth Cooper, Sharon Criss, Bonnie Friedman, Betsy Gilbert, Spencer Gilbert, Mare Kelley, David and Jana Ladner, Ruth Quimette, and Shirley Tuller.

The strength of this text lies in the nurse narratives. Ten practitioners graciously and enthusiastically told me their story. I am indebted to Anthony Adinolfi, Julie Barroso, Pat Cloonan Bonnano, Beth Black, Elizabeth Burkett, Susan Denman, Barbara Ezrig, Robin Moon, Ruth Quimette, and Shirley Tuller.

If this book is useful to students, it is due in large part to the careful and critical thinking of my editor, Elizabeth Tornquist, who again and again challenged me to take a fresh look at my approach to this effort. Without the endorsement and encouragement of Thomas Eoyang, my editor at W.B. Saunders, this book would not have come to fruition.

Finally, I am indebted to three women whose love and support have been as faithful as the seasons: Nancy Gilbert, Robin Moon, and Marianne Poldervaart.

Carolyn Cooper, PhD, RN

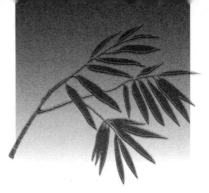

Contents

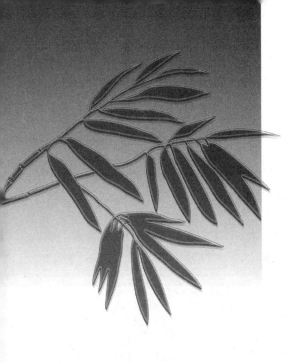

SECTION I

WHAT NURSES KNOW

....

The first section of this book looks at the kinds of knowledge you need to be an expert nurse. The book distinguishes between general or empirical knowledge, which comes from many sources and is widely accepted and available, and particular knowledge or knowledge that comes from the nurse, the patient, or the situation. These two forms of knowledge are used together by expert nurses to guide their response to patients.

Chapter 1 presents the stages through which students pass while acquiring both general and particular knowledge and nursing skills. Chapter 2 illustrates one type of particular knowledge known as personal knowledge in the story of Betsy, a geriatric nurse practitioner (GNP) working in a retirement community. The final chapter of this section focuses on the use of ethical knowledge. The story of David, a nurse working on a Bone Marrow Transplant Unit, illustrates the use of this knowledge, which is a combination of general and particular knowledge.

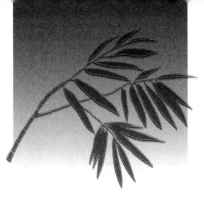

CHAPTER 1

Acquiring Nursing Knowledge

....

3

Introduction

The nurse working in the emergency room (ER) took one look at Tom and immediately set into motion the team's crisis response. The emergency medical technicians (EMT) who brought Tom in said that he had been in a work accident less than 30 minutes ago; he had lost one arm, and the other arm was badly damaged. Tom was conscious. His dark eyes, highlighted by the white sheets, were bright and piercing. *He knows he's in trouble,* the nurse was thinking as Tom spoke in a calm, clear voice: "I am a Jehovah's Witness. Do not give me any blood." Repeating this as a mantra, Tom stopped his entreaty only when the surgeon on call reassured him that the medical personnel would not give blood in surgery. Tom drifted into unconsciousness and was taken to the operating room (OR).

Eliese was the charge nurse in the surgical intensive care unit (SICU) to which Tom was brought after his surgery. Eliese received Tom from the OR transport team at 11:30 PM. The surgeon had not been able to save his other arm because of his low hematocrit (percentage of red blood cells) and poor perfusion. The tightly bandaged stumps that had replaced his arms struck Eliese. *He's so young,* she thought as she neatly arranged his intravenous and monitor lines. He was drowsy but easily aroused. His pain appeared to be moderate. As she took the report from the OR nurses, Eliese was told his condition was critical, in large part due to his low hematocrit. Eliese knew that without sufficient red blood cells to deliver oxygen to his vital organs, he could not survive.

"How much blood has he received?" she asked. "None," she was told. "He's a Jehovah's Witness and has refused a blood transfusion."

The patient was unstable and Eliese monitored him closely. About two in the morning, she received a call from the surgeon saying she had ordered two units of blood for Tom. Eliese protested, knowing that Tom had refused a transfusion. The surgeon explained that the patient's father, supported by Tom's wife, had made an impassioned plea to save Tom's life, even if it meant giving blood. The father had convinced the doctor to overrule Tom's decision not to receive blood.

Eliese was torn. She knew the transfusion could save Tom's life. Tom was 26 years old, a husband and father of two. He was so young, could he really know what he wanted? Eliese also understood the surgeon's perspective. After all, despite her best efforts, the surgeon had been unable to save Tom's arm, and now she was about to lose the patient.

Eliese went to Tom, whom she easily roused. "The doctor is telling me you need two units of blood. Do you want the blood?" she asked her patient. Intubated, Tom could not speak, but he shook his head, no. Eliese explained, "Tom, we could lose you if you don't get this transfusion. Do you understand what I am saying?" Tom nodded, indicating he comprehended what Eliese meant. He is alert and rational, Eliese thought. She asked one more time, "Tom, do you want the blood?" Tom shook his head, no.

Eliese called the surgeon and recounted her bedside conversation with Tom, saying he was refusing the blood and she would therefore not give it. Angry, the surgeon replied, "I'll come and give the blood myself if need be." Eliese held her ground, and the surgeon said, "I'll be right there."

Within ten minutes, the surgeon called again. Calmer now, she explained, "The whole team worked so hard to save this man. I keep thinking about his wife and children. It is hard not to intervene when a simple transfusion would probably pull him through." Nevertheless, she said that, like Eliese, she would honor Tom's wishes, despite the medical facts and the wishes of Tom's father and wife. She canceled the order for blood.

Reflecting on the experience, Eliese observed, "I could see where she was coming from, and she saw my position as well. Tom survived, but he could have died. He was willing to risk death because of his beliefs, and knowing that, both the surgeon and I honored his wishes."

General and Particular Knowledge

This vignette depicts the use by an expert nurse of two broad types of nursing knowledge—general and particular knowledge. General knowledge, that is, empirical or scientific knowledge, is widely used in health care. This body of knowledge includes knowledge about diseases, epidemiology, pathophysiology, anatomy, diagnosis, and treatment. The application of general knowledge, or objective knowledge, is straightforward; that is, the knowledge is applicable in much the same way to all patients. Eliese's general knowledge—for example, her understanding of physiology—made it clear to her that Tom's low hematocrit, reflecting his blood loss, meant reduced blood flow and oxygen to vital organs. She knew this could lead to his death. These principles of physiology would be true for all patients. The scientific knowledge you are learning in the classroom thus falls into the category of general knowledge.

Nurses rely heavily on general knowledge from many disciplines, including nursing and medicine, as well as the social and biological sciences. Indeed, general knowledge provides the foundation for understanding the physical, social, and psychological characteristics of individuals, families, and communities, and directs the nurse's assessment and interventions with patients. The explanatory and predictive power of general knowledge is pivotal in diagnosing and treating diseases. For example, Eliese and the surgeon understood that when Tom's hematocrit reached a certain percentage, without a transfusion he would probably die. Eliese's solid grasp of general knowledge was her starting point for practicing the art of nursing.

General scientific knowledge constitutes the basis for most nursing knowledge. Beginning in the late 1970s, however, nurse scholars noted that a profession that claimed to be both science *and* art could not rely exclusively on scientific knowledge. Carper (1978) argued that indeed, scientific knowledge overlooked the art of nursing or those subjective aspects of nursing that in large part define the profession. A similar argument was also being made in medicine. That is, both professions were beginning to recognize that general or scientific knowledge of patient diseases and treatments, while essential to diagnosis and management of the disease, overlooks the nonscientific knowledge of the patient's experience (Bartholome, 1992). This subjective knowledge can also be termed *particular knowledge.* Thus, relying upon her particular knowledge of Tom, Eliese was unwilling to give him blood when this contradicted his principles.

Particular knowledge is knowledge that is not generally known or applicable but is particular to the nurse, the patient, or the circumstances. This form of knowledge may be revealed by the patient to the nurse, or it may arise from the situation. Gadow (1995) calls particular knowledge of the patient "engaged knowledge," since it originates in part in an engagement or relationship between the nurse and the patient. Particular knowledge of the patient includes the patient's feelings and thoughts about illness, as well as the patient's values and goals (Bartholome, 1992). This particular knowledge may also include the patient's experience of pain or nausea; feelings such as fear, joy, or relief; or the patient's response to treatments and interventions. Particular knowledge also reflects the patient's response to applied general knowledge. For example, you will learn general knowledge about oxygen saturation, including the normal range for oxygen saturation in the blood. As you get to know particular patients, you will learn that some survive on levels of oxygen saturation that fall outside normal parameters. This applied general knowledge thus becomes a form of particular knowledge. Particular knowledge of the patient is the key to individualizing the nurse's response.

The nurse comes to the patient encounter with the general knowledge needed for the care of the patient, and the patient brings particular knowledge of himself or herself. The nurse must depend upon the patient or family members to convey relevant knowledge of the patient. In Eliese's story, Tom disclosed the information that he was a Jehovah's Witness and his values meant that he would choose possible death over a blood transfusion.

Both general and particular knowledge are needed to direct nursing interventions. Nurses need a solid grasp of the disease process, as well as an understanding of what illness means to the patient. Eliese relied upon general knowledge when she said to Tom, "We could lose you if you refuse this transfusion." Her particular knowledge of Tom's wishes and values led her to refuse the doctor's order to give the blood. Both forms of knowledge are central to the art of nursing. Incompetence in the form of a poor grasp of general knowledge or an unfeeling response to the patient when particular knowledge is ignored constitute a failure by the nurse. While one type of knowledge may take precedence over the other, as when Eliese urged the surgeon to honor Tom's refusal to receive blood, a firm grasp of both general and particular knowledge is a main ingredient in nursing.

Acquiring Nursing Skills

Ben took a deep breath and quickly dried his hands. A nurse for 12 years, he was working on a surgical floor. He had learned to calm himself when faced with an emergency by breathing deeply. Two days earlier his patient, Mrs. Floyd, had undergone surgery on her head and neck to remove a cancerous tumor. Aware of the risk of bleeding from the carotid, the major artery that supplies blood to the brain, Ben had just checked Mrs. Floyd's clean, white bandages looking for evidence of bleeding. He reassured the patient and her husband that everything looked good and then turned to wash his hands. Suddenly he heard Mrs. Floyd gasp. Instantly Ben thought, She's developed a carotid bleed.

He turned from washing his hands to see terror on Mrs. Floyd's face as blood spurted from her neck. Already the wall was splattered, and the pillow and sheets were drenched. Ben knew this was a life-threatening emergency. He knew the bleeding must be stopped, replacement blood sent for from the hospital blood bank, additional blood typed and cross-matched for surgery, and the operating room personnel and surgeon notified to receive Mrs. Floyd for repair of the carotid. He also knew Mr. and Mrs. Floyd's terror must be addressed.

An expert nurse, Ben was clear that the first task was to stop the bleeding. He stuck his head into the hall and shouted for help. Instantly other nurses on the floor responded. He directed while one nurse assisted him at the bedside, another headed for the blood bank to retrieve blood, and yet another escorted Mr. Floyd out of the room, reassuring him that the team was making every effort to get this crisis under control. In the room, gloved hands were everywhere, applying pressure to stop the bleeding, hanging fluids to replace Mrs. Floyd's rapidly declining fluid volume until the blood arrived, and preparing to transport the patient to the operating room.

Throughout the first minutes of the crisis, Mrs. Floyd's eyes searched the faces of the nurses for some clue as to what was happening to her, for some sign of reassurance. Within seconds after setting the team response into motion, Ben turned to her and without ceasing to direct what was happening in the room, said, "Mrs. Floyd, I know you are frightened, but we are working to get the situation under control. You are bleeding from your carotid artery. This happens sometimes after surgery such as yours. We're sending you back to the operating room to repair your carotid. You're in good hands. Your husband is with a nurse and he is fine. I will see you when you return from your surgery." Hearing his words, Mrs. Floyd visibly relaxed, closed her eyes and turned herself over to the team, who hurried her off to the operating room where her carotid artery was successfully repaired.

GENERAL ASPECTS OF SKILL ACQUISITION

In 1984 Patricia Benner wrote a classic book, *From Novice to Expert,* in which she described the progress of nurses as they master the skills of the profession. On the basis of observations and interviews with new nurses and expert nurses working together, Benner described five stages or levels of skill acquisition through which nurses pass. These levels of skill acquisition are mastered one at a time and in a particular order: 1. novice, 2. advanced beginner, 3. competent, 4. proficient, and 5. expert.

Ben's story depicts the expert nurse in practice. An indicator of his expertise was his ability to *interpret* the entire situation, zero in on what was most pressing, and act instantaneously. You will progress from being a novice nurse to an expert as you develop knowledge and nursing skills. Movement through the levels of skill acquisition requires clinical experience and practice. There is no substitute for experience on the journey toward excellence in nursing practice: reading about how to do something provides the foundation but cannot capture the expert's know-how (Benner, 1984). For example, knowledge of physiology can teach you what happens when patients bleed from the carotid artery. You can also learn from books the possible complications with head and neck surgery. However, no book can teach you how to instantly recognize the meaning of Mrs. Floyd's gasp—that she had a carotid bleed. Ben's understanding of this situation reflected the combination of a sound education, nursing judgment, experience in similar situations, and practice.

Three general aspects of skill acquisition characterize progress toward expertise in nursing practice. The first is a shift from relying on information learned in the classroom, to relying on concrete experience (Benner, 1984). You have already begun to make this shift if you have recognized that often there is a difference between what you learn from books and what you see in practice. For example, you have learned the parameters for administering pain medication; you know how much medicine can be given safely in a certain amount of time. In practice, however, you have probably learned that patients' needs may fall outside these parameters. Some patients need more medication than others do to control similar levels of pain. Other patients who have long-term pain develop a tolerance for pain medications and require doses far greater than those considered within normal ranges. Thus you will learn to rely on the patient's clinical picture, including physiological parameters, as well as what you know about the patient's tolerance of pain and response to medication to guide your administration of pain medications.

A second broad aspect of skill acquisition involves a shift from seeing aspects, or pieces of a situation, to seeing the situation as a whole and recognizing which aspects are relevant (Benner, 1984). As a novice nurse, you tend to focus on one thing at a time. If you are taking the patient's vital signs, you may not notice that the patient is pale and his lips have a bluish tinge. As you move from novice to expert, you will learn how to "take it all in" in a glance, as Ben did, and quickly focus on what is most important in the situation.

The third aspect of acquiring nursing skills is moving "from detached observer to involved performer" (Benner, 1984, p. 13). Until you master nursing skills, there will be an element of detachment in your delivery of nursing care; this is unavoidable since your focus must first be on *how* to perform the task. For example, when you are learning a skill like taking blood pressure, your focus necessarily is less on the patient and more on the steps you must go through to obtain the blood pressure. To learn the skill, your primary focus must be on the skill, not the patient. As you master skills, they will become second nature, enabling you to then engage with or assess the patient while performing the skill. For example, with practice, you will learn to take a blood pressure while also assessing the patient's physical and emotional responses.

NOVICE NURSE

The novice nurse is at the first stage of acquiring nursing skills. The nurse has had little hands-on experience and therefore has limited experiential knowledge. Lacking experiential knowledge, the novice relies heavily on rules and protocols. The novice nurse's responses therefore tend to be inflexible, and she has little ability to single out the most relevant nursing tasks to be performed (Benner, 1984). For example, recall the first time you took a patient's blood pressure, gave a shot to a patient, or did a sterile dressing change for a patient. Your focus was probably on the task at hand as you tried to remember all the steps in the procedure. At this early stage of skill acquisition, the novice cannot also notice other things, such as how the patient is tolerating the procedure. The challenge for the novice nurse is to prioritize, that is, to decide what feature of the situation requires immediate attention (Benner, 1984).

Let us imagine Ben as a novice nurse taking care of Mrs. Floyd. The scenario would have looked quite different (although with the help of experienced colleagues, the outcome for Mrs. Floyd would probably have been equally good).

Ben was washing his hands when he heard his patient, Mrs. Floyd, gasp. He turned to see a spurt of blood. Assuming from the amount of blood that this was an emergency, he wondered, What could have gone wrong? What should I do? He knew from what he had learned in nursing school that he had to stop the bleeding, but he had never before seen this much blood. Where is all that blood coming from? he asked himself. Could it be coming from her carotid? Yes, it must be the carotid, he tentatively concluded.

Rushing to the hall, Ben shouted, "Help." He then returned to his patient, quickly gloved, and began to put pressure on her neck with a large, clean towel. He wondered, Am I doing this right? Am I using enough pressure? Within seconds the other nurses on the floor were in the room. An experienced nurse took charge of the situation, setting in motion the team effort to get Mrs. Floyd on her way to the operating room for repair of her carotid.

As a novice nurse who had never seen a carotid bleed, Ben could not immediately interpret his patient's gasp, nor could he instantaneously put into place the multiple aspects of the complex life-saving intervention. Taking some time to think about what to do first, he decided to call for help. Then, based on the knowledge that massive bleeding quickly leads to death, he set about to stop the bleeding. This focus, while correct, was narrow. He could not coordinate the various demands of the situation. He could not see the terror on Mrs. Floyd's face or notice that her husband was still in the room. His responses were self-conscious (Benner, 1984), leading him to ask himself, Am I doing this right?

All expert nurses began as novice nurses. With some experience, the novice nurse moves to the level of advanced beginner. Ben, a novice nurse, helped the team. His anxiety was high, but he paid attention, learning all he could. He was on his way to becoming an advanced beginner.

ADVANCED BEGINNER

Benner's (1984) second stage of skill acquisition is advanced beginner. At this stage the nurse has gained some knowledge from experience but still retains a narrow focus on one or two aspects of a situation. For example, suppose you are in a clinical rotation in psychiatric nursing, working on a unit serving depressed patients. Your patient, who is usually quiet, begins to pace in the dayroom, occasionally hitting the back of a chair as he walks by. Your instructor points. "This is what agitation looks like. That patient is agitated." The next week, another patient suddenly gets up from lunch and begins to pace in the halls. You now can recognize the patient's behavior as agitated. Much of your time in clinical is spent learning to recognize such aspects of clinical practice (Benner, 1998). Still relying heavily on rules and focusing on only one or two aspects of a clinical situation, the advanced beginner cannot decide which aspects are most important or see the big picture in clinical situations.

A story recounted by Owen from his early nursing practice illustrates well the skills of the advanced beginner. A recent graduate, Owen had worked for six months on a medical-surgical floor in a midsized community hospital. He took his responsibilities seriously, read journals, and regularly returned to his nursing texts to reinforce his rapidly growing knowledge.

One day as Owen made rounds on his patients, he found Mrs. Wrenn, a 62-year-old woman who had recently undergone a total hip replacement, leaning forward in her bed and somewhat short of breath. He asked her if she was OK, to which she replied, "I'm fine." Owen noted that her skin was slightly clammy and her pulse and respirations had increased from the reading earlier in the day. Her blood pressure had dropped, though not a lot. Owen was not sure whether these findings were significant.

Despite her protests that she was fine, Owen decided that the clammy skin and changes in her vital signs were significant and needed further assessment. He asked an experienced nurse to come and examine Mrs. Wrenn. Upon entering the patient's room, this nurse quickly assessed her to rule out several possible explanations for her distress and left to call the physician. She had concluded that Mrs. Wrenn probably had a pulmonary embolus or clot in her lungs, requiring immediate intervention. Tests revealed that Mrs. Wrenn did indeed have a pulmonary embolus, and she was transferred to an intensive care unit for treatment and close monitoring.

As an advanced beginner, Owen was unable to take in all aspects of the situation and decide what this constellation of symptoms meant. He had never seen a patient with a pulmonary embolus. He did note, however, two aspects of the situation: the clammy skin and the change in Mrs. Wrenn's vital signs, and he knew these symptoms were significant in a postoperative patient. Owen's recognition of these two aspects of Mrs. Wrenn's condition was sufficient to send him to a more experienced nurse and probably saved Mrs. Wrenn's life.

COMPETENT

Benner (1984) suggests that after two to three years of experience in the same setting, the nurse is at the level of competence. Having learned from experience, the competent nurse prioritizes patient needs, deliberately plans, and is not easily distracted from the tasks and plans he has set out. The competent nurse can coordinate multiple and complex tasks while managing many different demands. Benner quotes a nurse describing this stage of skill acquisition:

> Now I come out of report and I know what their [patients] I.V.s [intravenous lines] are basically, and I have a couple of things that I know that I have to do. Before I go into the room, I write down what med I'm supposed to give for that day, and then

I'll walk in there and make sure that everybody's I.V. is fine. You go from bed to bed and just say hi, just introduce yourself. But I give them the message that I'm just attending to business. I check their I.V.s; I check their dressings. And then I feel fine. I know they're not going to bleed to death; I know that their urine output is OK; I know that their I.V.s are fine . . . then I have the whole morning set out and I can go ahead and do things. I am much more organized. [Benner, 1984, pp. 26–27]

The competent nurse has gained organizational skills and completes tasks more rapidly than the advanced beginner but lacks the speed and flexibility to recognize the meaning of situations and perform tasks that characterize the nurse at the next level of skill development, the proficient nurse.

PROFICIENT

At the fourth level of skill acquisition, Benner (1984) sees the nurse as proficient— at home with nursing skills. At this stage of development, having had more experience, the nurse's gaze has broadened to take in far more than one detail at a time in a situation. The nurse now recognizes when something does not look normal. "Whereas the competent person does not yet have enough experience to recognize the situation in terms of an overall picture or in terms of which aspects are most salient . . . the proficient performer considers fewer options and homes in on an accurate region of the problem" (Benner, 1984, p. 29). Having gained flexibility, the proficient nurse shifts readily from one plan to another, as patient needs dictate.

The nurse whom Owen called to assess Mrs. Wrenn was practicing at the level of proficiency. She simultaneously appreciated several features of Mrs. Wrenn's situation, focusing on the most important symptoms as she assessed the patient to rule out various possibilities. Her concentration was sharp when she noted significant symptoms and she understood the possible meanings of the cluster of symptoms.

EXPERT

At the fifth level of skill acquisition, the expert level, Benner (1984) suggests that the moment of hesitation, of considering a wide variety of options, is usually no longer necessary. Benner describes the expert as follows: "The expert nurse, with an enormous background of experience, now has an intuitive grasp of each situation and zeroes in on the accurate region of the problem without wasteful consideration of a large range of unfruitful, alternative diagnoses and solutions" (p. 32). The expert has highly developed perceptions and takes in all the relevant information, immediately comprehending what is important and setting in motion a plan of action. Benner wrote, "Capturing the descriptions of expert performance is difficult, because the expert operates from a deep understanding of the total situation; the chess master, for instance, when asked why he or she made a particularly masterful move, will just say: 'Because it felt right.' [Or] 'It looked good'" (p. 32). As an expert nurse, Ben simultaneously recognized what was going on with Mrs. Floyd and set in place complex and appropriate interventions that not only saved Mrs. Floyd's life but also recognized and responded to her personal feelings of terror.

Upon reading about these levels of skill development, students often wonder, Will I ever move beyond the early stages of the novice nurse or advanced beginner? and Will I practice safely at the early stages of skill acquisition? Remember that every nurse begins as a novice. Experienced nurses recollect their early days in nursing, and many are available to mentor and assist beginning practitioners. With help, experience, and commitment to the process, novice nurses will become experts.

Summary

Nurses rely upon two types of knowledge in practicing the art of nursing. The first is general knowledge, which is widely known and accepted as true. The second is particular knowledge of the patient and the situation. These types of knowledge are needed to practice artful nursing. However, knowledge alone cannot make an excellent nurse. Skills, which are developed in clinical practice, are the means by which the nurse uses what she knows. Patricia Benner's (1984) levels of skill acquisition illustrate the sequential stages through which all nurses pass as they move toward artful nursing.

References

Bartholome, W.G. (1992). A revolution in understanding: How ethics has transformed health care decision making. *ORB*, January, 6–11.

Benner, P. (1984). *From novice to expert.* Menlo Park, CA: Addison-Wesley.

Carper, B.A. (1978). Fundamental patterns of knowing in nursing. *Advances in Nursing Science, 1,* 13–23.

Gadow, S. (1995). Narrative and exploration: Toward a poetics of knowledge in nursing. *Nursing Inquiry, 2,* 211–214.

APPLICATION

....

ACTIVITY I
Group Discussion: Analysis of the Story

1. Imagine you are caring for Tom. What would you do when you received the order to give blood? What reasons would you give for your decision.

2. Now imagine you are working with Mrs. Floyd, the woman who suffered the carotid bleed. You are a student in your clinical rotation. You have called for help and the experienced nurses have taken over the case. You stay in the room to observe the nurses handle the crisis with Mrs. Floyd. What might you learn from watching these nurses (be specific)? How would your observation of the crisis contribute to your development of nursing skills?

ACTIVITY II
Case Analysis and Group Discussion: Identifying General and Particular Knowledge

You are a student nurse completing your first seven-week clinical rotation in a skilled nursing care facility. During this rotation you have grown particularly fond of Mrs. Wilson, a woman in her mid-70s who two years ago sustained extensive left-sided weakness following a stroke. Unable to care for her, her son placed her in the nursing home. The son is attentive to his mother, visiting her twice a week and often taking her out for a ride. You have talked with him several times, and he has told you that his mother taught school for many years and loved to garden. In turn, you have told Mrs. Wilson about your favorite schoolteacher, Mrs. Shaw, who let you read comic books each Friday afternoon. You have also brought Mrs. Wilson flowers from your garden on several occasions.

Mrs. Wilson suffers from contractures (shortening of the muscles) in her left arm and leg, making it impossible for her to stand or to sit straight in her chair. Her speech is halting and slow, and she is very hard to understand. Despite her limited ability to communicate and her bent posture, Mrs. Wilson always tries to look up at you when you arrive, offering a smile and reaching out her unaffected arm to you in greeting.

During this rotation you have bathed, positioned, turned, dressed, toileted, and fed Mrs. Wilson. You have also given her medications, taken her vital signs and blood pressure, rubbed her back, administered enemas, and moved her many times from bed to chair and back to bed. You have listened carefully as she explained the numerous family pictures in her room. You have told her about your own family and brought in pictures of your dog and your six-month-old nephew to show her.

At the conclusion of your rotation your relief at having successfully completed this first clinical rotation is tinged with sadness when you think of leaving Mrs. Wilson. You have worked closely with her. You know how much she looks forward to her son's visits and the weekly automobile ride with him. You know her favorite passages from her worn Bible, many of which you have read to her. You have learned just how to hold the spoon and how much to offer as you feed her so that she can swallow her food without choking. You also know that she prefers to start out sleeping on her right side and to wear socks when she sleeps.

As you say good-bye to Mrs. Wilson, you promise yourself that you will send her a card every now and then. Recognizing that the nurses and nursing assistants will not have the time to give her the attention you have provided, you carefully write out all you have learned about your patient and pass it along to the head nurse.

GROUP DISCUSSION QUESTIONS

1. Identify the general knowledge you have applied in your care of Mrs. Wilson.

2. Identify the particular knowledge you have about Mrs. Wilson.

3. Describe the sources of the general and particular knowledge you have about your patient.

4. Discuss what you see as the relationship between general and particular knowledge.

5. Discuss the relationship between your particular knowledge of Mrs. Wilson and your feelings of sadness.

6. The last assignment in your rotation reads as follows: "Complete a nursing assessment form comprising at least five questions to be used to access particular knowledge about the patient." What questions would you submit?

ACTIVITY III
Group Discussion: Acquiring Skills

1. Each member of the group should identify a skill or talent that you practice at the level of proficient or expert. These probably will not be in the area of nursing but might include academic areas in which you excel, such as chemistry; personal skills such as cooking or writing; or a hobby like playing chess, a musical instrument, or a sport.

2. Discuss how you developed this skill. Include the role of practice, your readiness to acquire the skill, and the role of a teacher in your discussion.

ACTIVITY IV
Self-Reflection: Identifying Particular
Knowledge of Yourself

1. Think about the story of Tom and Eliese. What would you have done if you had been the nurse? Why would you have chosen that course of action? What does your choice say about your level of skill acquisition?

2. Compare and contrast the differences between Ben as a novice and Ben as an expert nurse.

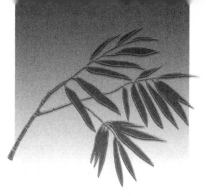

CHAPTER 2

Personal Knowledge

Introduction

Personal knowledge lies at the heart of nursing and provides the key to tailoring the nurse's response to the patient's needs. Personal knowledge is the knowledge nurses have of themselves and their patients (Sweeney, 1994). Personal knowledge also includes knowledge or mastery of nursing skills.

Personal knowledge is difficult to teach (Carper, 1978) because it is *personal,* making it impossible to apply it to everyone (Moch, 1990). This form of knowing is, however, familiar to all students. Everyone relies upon personal knowledge to guide behavior. For example, the knowledge you have about your reaction to stress dictates how you study for an examination. If you know that you tolerate pressure well, you may wait until the last hours to study; if you cannot endure last-minute cramming, you probably begin to study earlier.

This chapter opens with brief descriptions of three types of personal knowledge.
- Knowledge of yourself
- Knowledge of your patient
- Knowledge (mastery) of nursing skills

Knowledge of Yourself

Knowledge about yourself is gained from reflecting on your experiences. For example, when you live through and reflect upon ending an intimate relationship, you begin to learn the myriad feelings associated with such an experience. This self-knowledge can be useful to you in other close relationships.

The desire for self-knowledge is related to the need to become or to actualize one's unique self. This is no easy endeavor and involves challenging values and attitudes that simply reflect the values of others such as teachers, friends, or parents. As individuals mature, they incorporate some of these values and attitudes and reject others. This process of sorting out what is right for oneself or what simply reflects the expectations of others continues throughout life and rests upon truthfulness with oneself and reflection about one's behavior and responses. The opportunities for self-reflection are countless in nursing because of the multiple and varied interactions with patients. Seizing these opportunities is crucial to effective nursing because self-knowledge is the key to avoiding behaviors that may provoke feelings of anger, dependence, isolation, or frustration in patients.

There is a relationship between self-knowledge and effective nursing. When nurses are secure in the knowledge of who they are, they can accept patients as they are. For example, suppose your uncle is an alcoholic. As a child you noticed the negative effects of his drinking on himself and his family. Reflecting on this, you know that you have negative feelings toward persons with alcoholism. You gain self-knowledge when you recognize the origin of your negative feelings and can avoid letting negative feelings about persons with alcoholism influence how you respond to a patient who is an alcoholic.

Knowing herself also heightens the nurse's capacity to feel with the patient. That is to say, knowing her own feelings of sadness, joy, or fear enables the nurse to understand the same feelings in the patient. This is called empathy and is often the means by which nurses reach out emotionally to patients.

Knowledge of Your Patient

Personal knowledge also includes knowledge of the patient. Like self-knowledge, this knowledge comes from experience. General knowledge *about* patients is gleaned through the study of diseases and their symptoms, treatments, and effects. The applicability of this knowledge to a particular patient comes through reading the patient's chart. Knowledge *of* the patient includes knowledge of the patient's *response* to the disease, symptoms, or treatment, as well as how the patient's values impact on the illness experience (Jenks, 1993). This knowledge comes from the patient. For example, people respond to bad news differently. Some people remain quiet and calm when faced with setbacks, while others become anxious or depressed. The nurse needs to know the patient's response when faced with bad news to provide nursing care that is tailored to meet individual patient needs. Knowledge of how your patient feels about an illness or what your patient believes about health or who the patient feels close to—all of this is knowledge of the patient.

Nurses need this knowledge to individualize nursing care and to personalize standard nursing care plans or critical pathways. The knowledge is often gained by talking with and observing the patient or through conversations with family or close friends of the patient. Openness and acceptance make it easier to see the patient not as a diagnosis but as a complex and unique individual with particular needs.

Mastering Nursing Skills

Finally, personal knowledge involves the mastery of nursing skills, ranging from adeptness at giving injections to recognizing subtle changes in a patient's color. Like knowing oneself and knowing the patient, mastery of skills comes with experience. For example, you learn in the classroom that lung sounds change when a patient has congestive heart failure and these changes have meaning. This classroom knowledge about lung sounds becomes personal knowledge when you master the skill of hearing and interpreting lung sounds (Benner, 1984). This happens most easily when you listen to the lung sounds with an expert who points out their nuances and meaning. As you work with the expert, practice, and put this experience together with what you have learned in the classroom (Moch, 1990), gradually—or sometimes all at once—you "get it." The skill of hearing and understanding lung sounds has now become a part of your storehouse of personal knowledge.

How this actually happens is not easily explained. Philosopher Michael Polanyi (1958) illustrates the difficulty by describing the experience of learning to ride a bike. Someone who has mastered the skill of bike riding knows exactly how much to lean away from a curve to keep from falling over. But the subtleties of this know-how cannot be explained to a learner. No matter how much the novice biker reads about how to stay upright in a curve, mastery of the skill comes only as she watches other bikers and practices. The novice biker must get "a feel" for managing a curve. Then one day, with practice, the biker "gets it." The know-how of riding a bike becomes her own. Soon she no longer needs to think about how to stay upright—it has become natural. So it is with the mastery of clinical skills for the student of nursing.

Self-knowledge, knowledge of the patient, and mastery of skills are all illustrated by the story of Betsy, a geriatric nurse practitioner (GPN) working in a retirement community. Betsy's skillful management of her patient's congestive heart failure (CHF) extended his life by a year and a half. This story also illustrates the importance of recognizing one's own strengths and limitations in order to keep learning about oneself.

Betsy's Story

Mr. and Mrs. James were in their early eighties when they moved to a retirement community that served professional and relatively well-to-do retirees in a small university town. Both their son and daughter taught at the university. The family was close and included the daughter, who was unmarried, Bob Junior and his wife, and their children and grandchildren.

Betsy was one of two nurse practitioners in the retirement community. Her love of elderly patients had been kindled years earlier by her close relationship with her grandparents. What Betsy enjoyed most about elderly patients was helping them through the transitions of aging. She took pleasure in assisting them to remain independent as long as possible, using her own considerable skills as well as patient and family resources toward this end.

One day Mrs. James was admitted to the retirement community's health center with chills and fever. A chest x-ray confirmed a diagnosis of pneumonia. Betsy treated her pneumonia and also reviewed the management of her arthritis and diminishing vision, which, Mrs. James complained, were "slowing her down." Betsy found the patient a lively, petite woman who was well groomed despite her illness and held strong opinions about almost everything. Betsy also noticed that this woman was somewhat guarded in talking about herself, revealing little of how she felt.

On the morning after Mrs. James's admission, her husband arrived to check on his wife. A tall, large-framed man who was well dressed in an unassuming way, he conveyed a quiet confidence. After checking on his wife, Mr. James found Betsy. How was Mrs. James doing? he wanted to know. His soft-spoken manner took Betsy by surprise, given his great size. Betsy answered his questions and went with him to see Mrs. James.

Betsy noted that the couple appeared affectionate despite a formality in their interactions that she had often observed in older couples. Betsy reassured them that Mrs. James was doing well, and when she left, she invited Mr. James to stop and see her on her way out.

Mr. James and Betsy talked daily over the course of Mrs. James's five-day stay. Betsy noted, "One of the beauties of my job was the opportunity to talk with patients and get to know them well. This paid off handsomely because over time I learned how to figure out whether something was troubling patients just by observing their facial expressions." Less guarded than his wife, Mr.

James expressed his distress about his wife's illness. He was particularly worried about his ability to take care of her when she returned to the apartment.

As they talked, Betsy noted that Mr. James had some shortness of breath and slight swelling in his face and hands. He confirmed her impression that he had congestive heart failure (CHF). His condition greatly reduced his physical capabilities, he said, and he wished he could improve, if only minimally, his physical stamina.

In response, Betsy proposed that she review his medical records, call his physician, and the three of them work together to improve his fitness. He could start with mild fitness training in the physical therapy department of the retirement community. Enthusiastically Mr. James agreed. By the time Mrs. James was discharged to the apartment, Betsy had two new patients.

As was her custom, Betsy visited Mrs. James several times after her discharge to assess her adjustment to the home setting. On the morning of her third visit, as she entered the apartment, she noted on the stove a bright red, unattended, burning electric coil. There was no evidence anyone was cooking. Tactfully, Betsy said, "Mrs. James, I notice that the stove is on." Frightened by her carelessness, Mrs. James explained that she must have forgotten to turn the stove off and added that she couldn't see well enough to notice it was on. Betsy suggested that they paint red nail polish, which Mrs. James could see, on the markers indicating the off position. She then proposed that Mr. James double-check the stove after his wife cooked. This suggestion was met by a resounding "No" from both. Betsy backed off. She explained later, "They were right. They needed their work together to be complementary, not supervisory." Recognizing the danger of fire and Mrs. James' fear, Betsy continued to talk with her about ways she might have better control of the stove. Eventually, with full support from the couple, the stove was replaced with a microwave oven, and the couple increased their visits to the facility dining room.

As Mrs. James recovered, Betsy began to work more with Mr. James. Noting that he had been in the hospital several times with symptoms of CHF, she began to manipulate his cardiac drugs and diuretics to help him gain optimum benefit from them. This required close monitoring with frequent medication adjustments. Betsy would listen to his heart and lungs, attending closely to any unusual rhythm indicating delayed closure of the heart valve. She listened for crackles at the base of his lungs, and she felt his legs, checking for swelling. Depending on the complexity of his status, she would call his doctor for a consultation.

Betsy explained, "Despite everyone's best efforts, his CHF continued to progress. However, because I was able to talk with him about how he felt and listen to his heart and lungs regularly and adjust his medications, he did not ever have to go back to the hospital. Because of our close contact, I was able to pick up on the nuances of his status and adjust his medications accordingly. It was tricky since he had cardiorespiratory involvement as well as peripheral edema (accumulation of fluid), fluid in his lungs, and beginning kidney problems. I had to be careful not to tax his heart or his renal system with medicine. Adjusting his medications became a real balancing act."

While Mrs. James had revealed little about herself to Betsy, Mr. James increasingly talked to Betsy. Betsy said, "He began to trust me and talk to me." Betsy learned that Mr. James was an architect who had designed imaginative homes and public buildings. The couple had actually had three children, not two. Their firstborn son had inherited Mr. James' artistic ability and was following in his father's footsteps as an architect when he died in an automobile accident. Remembering his boy, Mr. James sobbed as he recounted the accident 25 years ago. He confessed that until this moment, wanting to protect his wife from his pain, he had never cried over his loss.

As time passed, Betsy saw a power struggle developing between Mr. James and his children, who did not want him to continue to drive because they felt he was no longer a confident or cautious driver. Insisting he was safe in his automobile, Mr. James said he needed to run errands in the car. The struggle reached a crisis when his well-meaning son took the spark plugs out. Mr. James figured out what had been done and was upset that his son had tried to trick him. He brought his concerns to Betsy, who was careful not to get caught in the power struggle and suggested she take a ride with him and his wife so the three of them could assess how he did. Betsy said, "I knew he was a wise man. I thought that if he actually drove with the intention of assessing how he managed, he would see for himself how difficult it was to drive with his slowed responses. I was going to call upon his wisdom to bring him to the conclusion that he should not drive. I hoped he could decide this for himself." The drive began in the parking lot, where Mr. James concluded, "I did OK, now let's tackle the roads." Slowly he drove the two women around the almost empty country roads, concentrating with great determination on the task at hand. Finally, he pulled the large, older model automobile into the parking lot, removed the key from the ignition, turned to his riding companions and announced, "I'm very glad to have had the opportunity to drive this car for the last time." Betsy noted,

"Like all of us, he needed to learn for himself. He realized that because of his slowed reaction time related to normal aging, compounded by the increasing shortness of breath related to his CHF, he could no longer safely manage driving and accepted this with grace."

Several months later the family celebrated the couple's 50th wedding anniversary in a tastefully decorated parlor at the facility. Mrs. James, at home entertaining, was decked out in a white silk suit complete with an orchid corsage, sent by her husband. Unable now to stand for long periods, Mr. James, looking his finest, sat with his two great-grandchildren on his lap to receive his guests while Mrs. James circulated among their friends.

Mr. James's CHF continued to worsen. Within weeks after the anniversary celebration, he could no longer leave his apartment without assistance. Soon he was requiring oxygen all the time. When Betsy suggested that he might be more comfortable in the Health Center where he could have assistance in meeting his needs, Mr. James said he wanted to remain in his home as long as he could. Once again Betsy resumed home visiting. She helped the couple convert the living room into a bedroom so Mr. James could sleep on the hide-a-bed couch and not disturb his wife, a poor sleeper, with his nighttime restlessness. Betsy found that managing his medications was increasingly complex. Despite her best efforts, his condition required frequent short stays in the Health Center.

As the weeks passed, Mr. James grew progressively weaker. At times his speech was limited by shortness of breath or he needed a longer period to recover from talking. Some days the swelling in his face or legs was greater, his lungs sounded wet from the fluid accumulating in his chest, or he could only breathe sitting up. Betsy would palpate his chest to feel for heaves and listen for adventitious lung sounds, noting what and where they were and what they meant. When he was especially short of breath, Betsy would help reposition him, gauging whether he could breathe better lying down or sitting up.

Sometimes Mr. James seemed preoccupied and simply stared out the window. Betsy would sit quietly with him or ask him, "What are you feeling? You are unusually quiet." In response, he would get a twinkle in his eye and reply, "You noticed, huh?" Then he would express fear that he might fall, or that he might not be able to catch his breath, or his wife would not be able to manage without him.

Two weeks before he died, Mr. James told Betsy he was ready to be admitted to the Health Center. Betsy knew this would be his last admission. She did not, however, speak directly to him about his approaching death. She explained, "I take my lead from the patient in regard to discussing death. He never indicated he wanted to talk about this with me, and I did not feel comfortable opening that conversation. After he died I wished that I had approached the topic with him just to see if he needed to talk about it, but I wasn't comfortable with that at the time. Now I have more self- and professional confidence. I would do it differently."

Mr. James' heart and kidneys were failing. He was increasingly short of breath and retaining fluid. Betsy told the family, who visited daily, that Mr. James was dying. As the last week of his life approached, he spoke infrequently and his restlessness increased. It seemed to Betsy that he was struggling against his death. She wondered if he was worried about how Mrs. James and his family would manage without him.

One morning the usually reserved Mrs. James wept as she said, "It is so hard on him. He is so restless. I wish there was something I could do to help him." Recognizing her need to help her husband, Betsy suggested, "Maybe he needs you to tell him that it is OK for him to go."

Mrs. James inquired, "Do you think that would help?"

Betsy replied, "I don't know, but we both know he is holding on for some reason. I know how much he cares about you and I know how much he wants things to be good for you after he is gone. He may need to hear from you that you will be OK. Do you feel you could tell him this?"

Accepting the challenge, she asked Betsy to come with her to Mr. James' room. With Betsy's encouragement, Mrs. James took her husband's hand and said, "Sweetheart, I'm OK. The children are all OK. You can let go when you are ready. We are all right."

Mr. James opened his eyes and looked at his wife with an intensity no one had witnessed in recent days. Then he closed his eyes. Mrs. James sat with him for a few hours and when she left she told Betsy that he seemed calmer.

Betsy left work early that day with an upper respiratory infection. That night, about ten o'clock, the nurse practitioner on duty called: "I think Mr. James will die tonight. His blood gases are bad. He is not responsive. Do you want to come in and see him?" Betsy said, "I knew she was probably right, that Mr. James was dying. I struggled with the decision. I was sick, but I knew it would not matter if he were exposed because he was dying. Yet I decided not to go in." Reflecting later on her decision to stay at home when the call came anticipating Mr. James' death, Betsy observed, "I think I did not go in part because of my immaturity as a nurse. I wasn't ready to let him go. I had helped the family say good-bye but I had not said good-bye myself." With some regret she added, "I would do that differently now. Now I would go without question. He trusted me. He trusted his safety with me. We had been through so much together that I feel I forfeited a real privilege for both of us."

Mr. James died that evening. Two days later Betsy attended his memorial service and visited Mrs. James, who at 84 was facing the prospect of living alone for the first time. Relying upon her family, friends, and Betsy for support, Mrs. James remained in her apartment for several years until her limited vision necessitated her move into the Assisted Living wing of the retirement facility.

Betsy concluded her story with a final thought about Mr. James. "He was ready with a smile; rarely did he need to be drawn out as we got to know each other. Basically he was a shy man—I am shy as well—and I think he felt I understood him. He could trust me with any information he wanted to share. I tried hard not to ever violate that trust."

Enacting Artful Nursing

Betsy's solid grasp of the pathophysiology of the cardiorespiratory system and the complex interplay of heart and lungs was key to managing Mr. James' medication regimen and extending his life. The art of her nursing lay in the way she combined this general knowledge with personal knowledge to respond to her patient's needs. Betsy's story illustrates her expert use of knowledge of herself and her patient, and her mastery of nursing skills. The following discussion focuses on three key nursing actions that illustrate Betsy's use of personal knowledge:

- Getting to know oneself
- Getting to know the patient
- Mastering practice skills

GETTING TO KNOW ONESELF

Knowledge of the self is gained by reflecting on life experiences. This requires courage and a willingness to look at one's behavior and learn from it. Students bring a wealth of self-knowledge to their practice. Some have positive and warm memories of being with and caring for grandparents. This experience may mean they enjoy older people, as was the case with Betsy. Others, who may have had less positive experiences with grandparents, may have concluded that they do not enjoy working with the older population. This acknowledgment is also a part of self-knowledge.

Betsy's story illustrates the use of self-knowledge to guide the nurse's response. Initially, Betsy went into geriatric nursing because she knew she enjoyed working with older adults. When she saw the stove burning red, she was tactful because she knew that the public exposure of a failing is embarrassing. When Mrs. James came to Betsy as Mr. James was dying, Betsy recognized in her what she knew well within herself—the need to be helpful and to relieve suffering. With this recognition in place, Betsy made her suggestion and then went with Mrs. James to talk to Mr. James. Betsy also acknowledged her own and Mr. James' need to "learn things for ourselves" when she arranged to go with Mr. James to help him assess his driving abilities.

Betsy's story demonstrates the ongoing process of getting to know oneself. As she recalled her care of Mr. James, Betsy asked herself why she did not speak directly with him about his impending death. Betsy said that she "did not feel comfortable opening that conversation." But she later concluded, "Now I have more self- and professional confidence. I would do it differently." Betsy's choice at the time represented a lost opportunity for both Betsy and Mr. James since she felt he might have needed to talk about his death. However, she transformed the lost opportunity into a chance to learn about herself. Her knowledge that she was not comfortable in this territory became the impetus for pushing her own boundaries and growing. The next time, in a different situation, Betsy would be prepared to "do it differently."

Reflecting on her choice not to go to Mr. James when he was dying, Betsy also came to realize that she did not go in part because she had not said her good-byes to this patient and did not want to let him go. Acknowledging that while she could help the family say good-bye but could not do so herself, she concluded, "I have better skills at self-care and I would go without question . . . I forfeited a real privilege for both of us."

Betsy's courage in her self-appraisal, which included recognizing lost opportunities and failures, is important to continued learning about the self. In her maturity, Betsy had come to recognize that the nurse-patient relationship is not unlike other relationships. There are occasions when the nurse is not there for the patient, or the nurse makes a judgment about what to say or not to say that she later regrets. Betsy accepted the limitations and strengths of her responses to Mr. James and, recognizing the ongoing process of developing self-knowledge, learned what she could from them.

GETTING TO KNOW THE PATIENT

Building upon her broad understanding and years of experience as a nurse, Betsy grounded her responses to the Jameses in personal knowledge of the couple. Her fundamental acceptance of her patients, evident in her receiving the guarded Mrs. James with the same welcome she extended to Mr. James, who was more open, set the stage for her work with the couple.

Betsy's efforts to get to know both Mrs. James and Mr. James were numerous. She invited them to talk with her and made visits to their apartment, listening carefully to what they told her and responding to what she heard. For example, early on Betsy took note of Mr. James's wish to improve his physical stamina and suggested he begin a modest program of strength training. Later, when Mr. James was dying, Betsy heard Mrs. James's wish that she could "do something to help him" and used this opportunity to guide Mrs. James through the process of telling her husband good-bye.

As Betsy got to know the Jameses, she became a sounding board for Mr. James and finally Mrs. James, enabling Mr. James to release his long-held grief over his son's death and Mrs. James to say good-bye to her dying husband. She helped the family resolve their conflict over Mr. James' continued driving. Acknowledging Mr. James' wish to stay at home as long as he could, she helped them reconfigure the apartment so Mr. James could sleep in the living room and not disturb his wife's fitful sleep.

Betsy understood that patients know more about themselves than the nurse can ever know. She trusted Mr. and Mrs. James to reveal what was important. Further, as she came to know Mr. James, she learned to trust his wisdom, helping him figure out for himself whether he should continue to drive. With Mrs. James, whom she knew less well, Betsy was more directive. When Mrs. James came to Betsy as Mr. James was dying, Betsy said: "Maybe he needs you to tell him it is OK for him to go . . . do you feel you could tell him this?"

It is not always clear how to respond. Sometimes cues are missed or misinterpreted. Recall Betsy's recommendation that Mr. James check behind his wife to be sure the stove was off. The couple responded with a resounding "No!" Recognizing that she had missed a significant aspect of their relationship, Betsy immediately backed off. However, in her retreat she did not ignore the potential problem with the stove. She continued to talk with Mrs. James and helped the couple see that they needed to disconnect the stove.

MASTERING PRACTICE SKILLS

Betsy's skills in physical and psychological assessment illustrate yet another aspect of personal knowledge. When Betsy listened with her stethoscope to Mr. James's heart and lungs, she heard the nuances of change in the familiar rhythms and sounds. When she palpated his legs for edema or his chest for heaves, or touched his skin to note whether it was damp or dry, the knowledge she needed to assess the patient was in her hands. Her skilled observations enabled her to note changes in his skin color, his breathing patterns, or the use of the accessory muscles in his chest to breathe. She noted how long it took him to recover his breath after speaking and whether he needed to be upright to catch his breath or could be comfortable lying down. Furthermore, she knew the meaning of these observations. She observed his pensive look and asked, "What are you feeling?"

Betsy's education as a nurse practitioner, coupled with years of practice, gave her a large store of knowledge that enabled her to respond to the patient as a unique individual, not as a faceless form. At the conclusion of her story, in answer to the question, "How did you gain your knowledge?" Betsy responded, "I started my learning in the classroom. Then with practice, experience, and working side by side with some excellent mentors, my knowledge began to grow. Initially my formal education was key; later experience played the larger part."

Challenges to Personal Knowing

As a nurse you will have multiple opportunities to get to know yourself. When interactions with patients are chaotic or difficult, it is your responsibility to examine the impact of your behavior upon the relationship. This is difficult, requiring personal courage and time for reflection. A counselor, if needed, or a wise and trusted friend can facilitate this. Self-scrutiny also requires that the nurse extend to herself an attitude of acceptance and nonjudgment. Recall how Betsy looked without self-blame at what she called her "immaturity as a nurse." She examined her behavior with the intent of learning about herself. Extending to herself the same acceptance and compassion she offered her patients contributed to her growth as a nurse.

A second way to gain self-knowledge is to tell your nursing stories. Betsy came to new self-understanding about her comfort in "pushing the boundaries" with patients as she told her story about Mr. and Mrs. James. As you tell your stories, it will be easier to see the action and learn about yourself.

Two major restrictions in getting to know the patient are time and technology. Unlike Betsy's work setting, in most acute care settings there is no time to get to know patients as Betsy came to know Mr. and Mrs. James. However, in some nursing specialties such as rehabilitation, management of HIV, renal dialysis, or long-term care, the patient's condition dictates frequent nurse-patient encounters, and with more patient contacts there are more opportunities to get to know the patient. Regardless of the nursing specialty, all nurses are pressed for time and in most settings nurses find themselves with too many patients and too little time to talk with each person.

This problem can be confronted in several ways. First, as your technical skills improve, you will learn how to talk with the patient while you do an assessment or provide treatment. You will also learn how to zero in on what is important to your patient so you can elicit the personal information you need to give good care. And you will learn how to get to know patients through observation. You can notice how the patient tolerates pain or reacts when the family comes to visit, or what makes the patient anxious, or what soothes the patient. When time is extremely limited, you can simply ask a patient, "What are your concerns about this situation and how can I help you?"

Technology can also impede getting to know the patient. Technology dominates many specialties and at times overshadows the patient. For example, the machines in intensive care or dialysis units are noisy, imposing, and demanding. They beep, squawk, and chirp, communicating to the nurse in a louder and more persistent voice than that of the patient. It is easy in these situations to look to the technology for knowledge *about* the patient and overlook personal knowledge *of* the patient. Perhaps the most useful antidote to this is to consciously recall personal knowledge of yourself—what it feels like to be scared, lonely, or sick. This self-remembrance is an excellent means for understanding the patient.

It is also difficult to get to know patients when they are too ill to talk or don't want to be known by the nurse. In these circumstances, knowledge of the patient is limited to what can be learned from family members or by observing the patient. Using Betsy's response to the guarded Mrs. James as a model, students can learn how to honor patients' reluctance to talk about themselves while remaining open and attentive to possibilities for connection with patients when they arise.

Finally, for a variety of reasons, nurses sometimes do not like a patient. This naturally leads to a reluctance to get to know the patient. In these situations, acknowledgment of your negative feelings about the patient is a prerequisite to choosing to provide excellent nursing care despite your feelings.

Opportunities to master practice skills are built into nursing programs. Students practice in skills labs and then with their instructor or preceptor in clinical settings. However, in some clinical situations there may not be enough learning opportunities to go around. Everyone does not get to catheterize a patient or start an intravenous line. In these circumstances, you can focus on learning the theoretical foundations for the skills—anatomy, physiology, and sterile technique—so you will be ready when the opportunity to practice arises.

Some students struggle with internal constraints to developing practice skills. Fear of or discomfort with being watched by the teacher may dampen enthusiasm about working with complex patients or volunteering for practice opportunities. Knowledge of one's fear, coupled with a supportive colleague who offers encouragement, will go a long way toward overcoming the reluctance to take on the challenges inherent in the practice of nursing skills.

Summary

The development of personal knowledge requires an intention to learn along with what Polanyi (1958) calls a passionate investment of energy in the experience. You will begin to generate and use personal knowledge in your practice as you pay attention to what is happening in clinical practice, consciously tie classroom knowledge to clinical practice, reflect upon and talk about your experiences, and watch experts in practice. This process will be helped along as you read stories about expert nurses such as those in this text. Finally, development of personal knowledge will be supported by openness to seeing what has not been seen or understood before (Sweeney, 1994). Of course, you must practice, practice, practice.

References

Benner, P. (1984). *From novice to expert.* Menlo Park, CA: Addison-Wesley.

Carper, B.A. (1978). Fundamental patterns of knowing in nursing.

Gadow, S. (1990). Response to "Personal knowing: Evolving research and practice." *Scholarly Inquiry for Nursing Practice, 4,* 167–170.

Gadow, S. (1995). Narrative and exploration: Toward a poetics of knowledge in nursing. *Nursing Inquiry, 2,* 211–214.

Jenks, J.M. (1993). The patterns of personal knowing in nurse clinical decision making. *Journal of Nursing Education, 32,* 399–406.

Moch, S.D. (1990). Personal knowing: Evolving research and practice. *Scholarly Inquiry for Nursing Practice, 4,* 155–166.

Polanyi, M. (1958). *Personal knowledge.* Chicago: University of Chicago Press.

Sweeney, N.M. (1994). A concept analysis of personal knowledge: Application to nursing education. *Journal of Advanced Nursing, 20,* 917–924.

APPLICATION

··

ACTIVITY I
Group Discussion: Analysis of the Story

1. Betsy decided not to return to the retirement community when Mr. James was dying. What would you have done if you had been in her situation? What are the reasons for your decision?

2. Mr. James was dying and needed Betsy. Betsy was ill and needed to stay at home. Discuss how the nurse balances the tension between patient needs and the needs of the nurse. What do you think are the limits to caring for others? When is it right to put your needs ahead of the patient's needs?

3. What did Betsy mean when she said that by not going back to be with Mr. James when he died she failed herself and her patient?

ACTIVITY II
Group Discussion: Developing
Personal Knowledge

If you have completed the workbook section in Chapter 1, recall the activity that you identified in Activity II, Question 1. If you have not completed this section, refer to Chapter 1, Activity II, Question 1, to identify a personal activity in which you excel. Within the group, each person in turn should again reveal the activity in which she is proficient or expert. Now, as a group, discuss the following questions as they relate to this activity:

1. How did you develop this skill?

2. How long did it take you?

3. If you had a formal or informal teacher who helped you learn this skill, describe your relationship to your teacher.

4. What was the role of practice in your development of the skill?

5. What was it like the first time you tried to do what you now do at a proficient or expert level?

6. What is it like for you now when you practice this skill?

7. How does mastery of this skill relate to the mastery of nursing skills?

ACTIVITY III
Case Analysis and Group Discussion: Developing Self-Knowledge

You are the nurse caring for a young married woman who has had emergency surgery for a bowel obstruction. Her husband is extremely anxious and refuses to leave her room. He questions everything you do for the patient and demands an explanation for every aspect of her care. Whenever you ask the patient a question, he immediately jumps in and answers for his wife. She accepts this behavior without questioning it. You soon began to avoid going into the patient's room.

1. What feelings does this situation evoke in you?

2. Can you relate this man's behavior or the response of his wife to anything in your own experiences? If so, describe that experience.

3. How could you use this situation to develop knowledge about yourself?

4. How might this self-knowledge help you in your responses to this patient, her husband, and other individuals with similar characteristics?

5. Discuss how the nurse develops self-awareness.

ACTIVITY IV
Self-Reflection: Learning About Myself

In the space provided, complete the following statements as they relate to aspects of yourself:

1. I would describe myself in regard to personal traits as

2. The personal characteristics that I like about myself and that I bring to my career as a nurse are

3. The personal characteristics that I do not like about myself and that I bring to my career as a nurse are

4. The characteristics that I admire most in some nurses are

5. My goals in regard to developing these characteristics for myself include (be specific)

6. The characteristics that I do not like in some nurses are

7. I think some nurses behave in ways that are not helpful to patients because

8. The patient characteristics that are most likely to be upsetting to me are

9. The patient characteristics described in question 8 are likely to upset me because

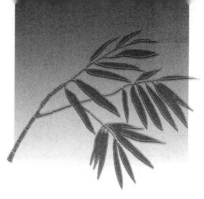

CHAPTER 3

Ethical Knowledge

Introduction

Ethics is the study of what is right or good. Ethical nursing practice is based on general knowledge about ethical frameworks and principles, professional codes and guidelines, and particular knowledge of one's values and the values of the patient. Knowing about ethics, however, is not the same as developing an ethical nursing practice. Moving from knowing about ethics to being an ethical nurse is similar to developing any other nursing skill. What is required is an intention to learn, self-reflection about values, the conscious integration of ethical knowledge with practice dilemmas, a skillful teacher, dialogue with others, and practice.

This chapter highlights three topics related to ethical knowledge that comprise a beginning framework for building an ethical practice:

- The ethical obligations of nurses
- Ethical frameworks and principles
- Values affecting nursing practice

The Ethical Obligations of Nurses

Because nursing actions have the potential for harm or good, they have a strong ethical component. Several characteristics of nursing impose upon nurses the obligation to do good. First, nurses work with people who are ill and vulnerable. Illness limits the capacity to care for oneself and the freedom to come and go as one pleases. Further, most patients are strangers in a health care system with its bizarre technology and unfamiliar language. Their experiences with health care add to their vulnerability. The obligation to alleviate this vulnerability is a chief attribute of nursing.

A second basis for the ethical obligations of the profession is the direct relationship between the nurse's actions and the patient's well-being. If the nurse is incompetent, the patient may die. If the nurse is callous about the patient's needs, the patient will feel diminished. Alternatively, if the nurse is competent and responsive to the patient's needs, the patient will feel safe and affirmed. This impact of the nurse on the patient heightens the obligation to do good.

Nurses' ethical responsibility is underscored by the public trust in nurses. Patients expect the nurse to act in their best interest. This expectation is met with an unspoken promise made by the nurse when she joins the profession—a promise that she will take care of patients.

The need to alleviate patient vulnerability, the direct impact of nursing actions on patients, and the public trust in nurses impose special ethical obligations upon members of the profession.

Ethical Frameworks and Principles

The nurse needs to know ethical frameworks and principles to build an ethical practice. Until the 1980s, nurses primarily used two ethical frameworks—deontology and teleology. Deontology describes an approach to action that is based on one's duty to follow certain ethical imperatives or mandates. For example, suppose a wealthy potential hospital benefactor is among your patients. You are asked to give her special treatment, even at the possible expense of failing to provide excellent care to other patients because there is a strong possibility that she will make a large bequest to the hospital that can be used to expand services to the poor. You are a deontologist; you follow certain ethical imperatives, including the imperative to treat all persons equally, according to their needs. Therefore, you take excellent care of the potential benefactor, but you do not give her special treatment beyond the care you provide for all patients.

The ethical framework of teleology would lead to a different response. According to this framework, the rightness of action depends upon the consequences or outcomes of one's behavior. Once again suppose the wealthy potential hospital benefactor is among your patients. You are a teleologist; you support special treatment beyond your usual excellent care to this patient since the money donated by this satisfied patient-benefactor will expand hospital services to the poor and result in a great good for many persons. This might mean that you would put this patient's needs above other patients' needs because you believe that the end (expanded services to the poor) justifies the means (special treatment to one patient, even at the possible expense of other patients).

Since the late 1980s, the ethic of care described by Gilligan (1982) has been used as an ethical approach by many nurses (Davis, 1986; Huggins & Scalzi, 1988). Within this ethical framework, right action is determined not by preestablished ethical imperatives or a focus on outcome but by needs that arise within a caring relationship. Engaging with patients, promoting the welfare of patients and family, and meeting the needs of all are paramount. Within this framework, the response of the nurse is based on patient circumstances that are revealed in the nurse-patient encounter. As patient needs change, the nurse's response changes, but the involvement of the nurse with the patient remains constant. From the framework of an ethic of care, your response to the potential hospital benefactor would be driven by the needs of the patient as they arise within the nurse-patient encounter. Your primary concern would be to meet all your patients' needs without a potential benefit to the hospital in mind or a sense of duty derived from an abstract ethical principle.

Ethical principles are abstract statements that help to guide ethical behavior. The following principles are particularly important for nursing practice: autonomy, truthfulness, beneficence, confidentiality, fidelity, and justice. Autonomy means self-rule (Yeo & Moorhouse, 1996, p. 92). Autonomous patients are self-determined and play a key role in making decisions related to treatment and care. Information is central to the ability to make autonomous decisions. In situations when patients cannot actualize their autonomy, family members or surrogate decision-makers who speak on behalf of patients should make every effort to honor what the patient would want.

Truthfulness entails not misleading the patient. Patients cannot be autonomous in decision making without a realistic understanding of their medical condition. Nurses may mislead patients by directly lying to them, by not giving enough information to enable an informed choice, or by not answering questions or failing to tell the patient who can provide needed information.

Beneficence means to do good and "requires us to act in a way that benefits others" (Yeo & Moorhouse, 1996, p. 58). Most health care professionals want to do what is good or right on behalf of patients. However, it is not always easy to know what constitutes good or right action. Ideally, the patient determines perceptions of good, and these are supported by the nurse, but in some situations this does not occur, and patients' wishes are overruled by nurses and physicians.

Confidentiality means not disclosing private patient information to unauthorized individuals. The nurse does not reveal the identity of patients to any individual who is not directly involved in the patient's care. Confidentiality is critical to patient trust and willingness to share private details related to health issues with the provider.

Fidelity means faithfulness. There are no ethical justifications for abandonment of a patient. In circumstances when the nurse feels she cannot provide good care for a patient, the nurse is obligated to get someone else to assume care of the patient.

Justice has various meanings but in a basic sense it has to do with fairness in determining "what someone or some group is owed, merits, deserves, or is otherwise entitled to" (Yeo & Moorhouse, 1996, p. 212). Issues of justice are broadly related to the fair distribution of health care resources and individually associated with decisions about how nurses allocate their time, for example, to multiple patients.

Ethical principles help the nurse make choices in ethical dilemmas. An ethical dilemma occurs when a person "believes that, on moral grounds, he or she both ought and ought not to perform act X" (Beauchamp & Childress, 1989, p. 5). For example, recall the case in Chapter 1. Eliese was caring for a man who was a Jehovah's Witness and had refused the blood transfusion needed to save his life. Against the man's wishes, the doctor ordered Eliese to give him blood. Eliese made an ethical argument for withholding the blood on the basis of the principle of patient self-determination. An equally strong ethical argument could have been made to administer the blood to save the patient's life on the basis of the principle of beneficence or doing good. Indeed, Eliese herself was torn between these two positions. Ethical dilemmas are daily fare in nursing practice.

Values Affecting Nursing Practice

Because nursing is ethical, values play a prominent role in nursing practice. Often the nurse must balance the values of the profession with personal and patient values.

The professional values of nursing are set out in documents such as Nursing's Social Policy Statement, published by the American Nurses' Association (ANA) (1995), and the ANA Code of Ethics with Interpretive Statements (1997). Nursing's Social Policy Statement describes the relationship of the profession to society and the professional obligations to those who receive care. Defining nursing as the "diagnosis and treatment of human responses to actual or potential health problems" (p. 6), this document mandates an approach to patients that attends to the full range of human experience and includes "practices that are restorative, supportive, and promotive" (p. 11).

The ANA Code of Ethics (1997) delineates ethical requirements for nurses and describes "the moral obligations and duties of every individual who enters the nursing profession" (p. 1). The code emphasizes the role of compassion, respect, and commitment in patient care. Stressing regard for the dignity of all patients, the code insists that patient values direct nursing responses and overrule the values of the nurse when there is a conflict.

Personal values also influence your ethical practice. As a student, you bring a wealth of knowledge about ethics to your practice, knowledge derived from formal study of ethics, religious education, parental injunctions, your own life experiences, and depictions of ethical behavior in the arts and literature. This knowledge is translated into personal values through experiences that test what you have been taught. For example, your parents may have told you long ago that "honesty is the best policy." As a nursing student you take an examination for which you are not prepared. During the examination you cheat by copying your neighbor's answers. Later you feel that you have betrayed your friend and yourself by using answers that were not your own. As a result of your discomfort, you decide for yourself that honesty is the best policy. The value of honesty, taught by your parents, is now your own.

Personal values are important because they are the starting point for ethical behavior and personal integrity. When someone has integrity, he or she acts from a position of ethical self-determination or autonomy (Yeo & Moorhouse, 1996). There is no need to rely upon others to determine the right thing to do. Rather, the person assumes control over and accountability for his own behavior. The ethically autonomous nurse does not falsify charts; she does not make this choice because she fears getting caught or because her nursing instructors taught her not to misrepresent records but, rather, because she believes it is wrong to lie.

Another characteristic of someone with integrity is that he is faithful to promises made, or true to his word (Yeo & Moorhouse, 1996). Fidelity supports patient trust and is essential to effective encounters between nurses and patients. When a nurse has integrity, he does not abandon a patient but continues to provide care, even when the patient has refused further treatment and is dying. Faithfulness to promises also means that the nurse follows through when she tells a patient that she will "be right back."

A final feature of integrity is that the nurse stands fast and speaks up for what is right (Yeo & Moorhouse, 1996). In illness, the nurse's advocacy for the patient creates a safe climate that supports healing. Speaking up for patients may be as easy as getting sufficient pain medication for a patient or as difficult as standing up for a competent patient who refuses life-saving surgery.

Patient values are always relevant in health care decisions, but patients' values are not always known. In some situations patients are too ill to express their wishes and there are no known family, friends, or written directives to inform health care decisions. In other cases, patients are so overwhelmed by illness and the health care system that, if no one helps them, they are unable to articulate their wishes. There are also situations when patients' wishes are known but ignored. Helping patients clarify what they want in relation to treatments and other health care decisions is a significant feature of ethical nursing. This is part of the role of the nurse as advocate and is more fully described in Chapter 5, Advocacy for Patients.

When patient values or wishes are known and compatible with the values of the nurse or health care system, they are easy to support. It is more difficult to support patient values when they conflict with the values of the nurse. In these cases, the professional values of nursing are useful as a guide to nursing action. For example, you may believe that individuals whose cigarette smoking or IV drug use has led to their illness do not deserve the same quality of care as persons whose illness is not related to lifestyle choices. You may not feel compassion for such patients and may wish to neglect them or even refuse to care for them. However, the American Nurses' Association (ANA) Code of Ethics (1997) says that the nurse must practice "with compassion and respect for the inherent worth and dignity of every individual . . . irrespective of the nature of the health problem" (p. 3). In cases of conflict, these professional values override personal values.

There are also situations in which the patient's values, as well as your own values, may conflict with professional values. For example, your patient may be dying a protracted death. The patient asks you to please give her an overdose of pain medication that would "take her out." You share your patient's wish for an easy death over a prolonged death. However, professional values dictate that nurses do not participate in active euthanasia. Thus, you must refuse to honor the patient's request to hasten her death.

The ethical nature of nursing, the role of values, and the complexity and uncertainty in ethical struggles are illustrated in David's story. Guided by the principles of patient autonomy and beneficence and the framework of the ethic of care, David's struggle was to determine the needs of his patient, Chip, and to balance Chip's needs with those of his wife, Lois.

David's Story

Chip was a handsome business executive in his forties; he loved to read and talk about ideas but mainly cherished time with his wife and two teenage boys. One day he went to his doctor complaining of a low-grade fever and aching in his knees and thighs. Routine lab work revealed that Chip had chronic myelogenous leukemia (CML), a blood disorder that is eventually fatal. While Chip could get a remission with medications, the only lasting cure was a bone marrow transplant (BMT).

An optimist, Chip proclaimed that he would beat the illness. He began a six-month course of oral medications to control the proliferation of the white blood cells and get his disease into remission. During this time Chip felt relatively well and continued his normal activities—working, spending time with his family, and going to church.

After six months, Chip was referred to the regional medical center for a BMT. David, a seasoned nurse working in the BMT unit, met Chip and his family during Chip's initial workup. David immediately liked this family, all of whom were curious, bright, and optimistic yet evidencing a vulnerability befitting the gravity of the situation. "Bone marrow transplants are not easy procedures," David explained later. "They cause extreme suffering. I try to help patients through that experience."

Chip was a fine candidate for a successful transplant and a full recovery. He was young, strong, had excellent insurance and financial resources, and had a loving and supportive family. Everyone expected a good outcome.

It was decided that Chip's 13-year-old son, Alan, would donate the marrow. The match was not perfect but was good enough. David explained, "A perfect match is much better because it reduces the chances of developing graft versus host disease (GVHD) or graft rejection, both of which can lead to mild or severe complications. I assess carefully for any sign of GVHD, a condition in which the T cells in the donor marrow attack the patient's body. GVHD can kill a patient."

When David admitted Chip to the busy BMT unit, he reviewed the treatment protocol and explained the rigors and side effects of the radiation and chemotherapy to be used to eliminate the disease and make a space for the transplanted marrow (ablative therapy). He explained that the treatment would require three to four weeks of hospitalization. Chip would be in seclusion most of that time while waiting for the bone marrow transplant to "take." "It is not easy," he told Chip. He urged Chip to take pain medications whenever he needed them and asked Lois to bring in Chip's own freshly washed clothes and some family photos to offset the drabness of the hospital gowns and the impersonality of the small private room.

David then asked Chip how he felt about the treatment. David said, "I always ask patients this. It sets the tone for our relationship by letting them know they can talk to me about whatever is on their mind, including their feelings." Chip's optimism was reflected in his response: "I feel like this experience is a wake-up call for all of us. I believe something good will come out of this if we work along with it." Chip asked David to keep him informed and teach him whatever he could. Agreeing, David turned to Lois and asked, "How are you doing?" With what David interpreted as a forced smile, she replied, "I'm ready to lick this thing." Then she added, "I simply could not carry on without Chip."

The next morning Chip began the ablative therapy while Lois transformed his room. She placed family pictures on a table and Chip's growing collection of cards, along with a large banner from church members that read "Get Well Soon, We Love You," on the wall. Lois also brought a small, framed, cross-stitched message that read, "Today is the first day of the rest of your life." She propped this on the chest that held Chip's clothes.

Chip's sons visited daily. David recalled Alan, the marrow donor, as a typical 13-year-old whose cap sat backward on his head. Dressing much like David's teenage son, Alan wore his boxer underwear three inches higher than his too large jeans that hung precariously on his slim hips.

One afternoon David found Alan alone and used this occasion to ask if he had any concerns about serving as a donor for his father. Alan shook his head: "It's no big deal, I just want Dad to get well." He shifted from foot to foot as if uncomfortable with David's query. David touched his shoulder and wished him luck.

Each day David talked with Chip about his treatment, books, movies, the challenges of teenage boys, and even religion. He came to know Chip as a deeply religious person whose concern for his family's well-being was primary regardless of how he felt. Chip talked to his boys on the phone daily and worried about Alan having to go through the bone marrow donation. He was also attentive to Lois, whose dependence on Chip was becoming more evident as the days passed. Making the two-hour commute to the medical center, Lois arrived early each morning and stayed all day. David would urge her to leave to get meals and some fresh air, but mostly she spent her time holding Chip's hand or sitting quietly reading.

David's routine included frequent checks on his patients. Late one morning he knocked gently and walked into Chip's room. Quickly Chip's finger went over his mouth to indicate silence. Lois was asleep, her chair pulled close to the bed, her head resting near Chip's sheltering arm. David was deeply touched to see Chip's protective gesture. Quietly he backed out of the room.

When the ablative therapy was complete, Chip received Alan's donated marrow. The wait began for the anticipated climb in his blood counts, which would indicate that Chip was making his own cells. To help Chip and Lois chart Chip's progress, David wrote the results of each day's lab work on a large, calendar that faced the foot of Chip's bed. David said, "This is normally the toughest time in the process. The wait is literally a matter of life or death. Patients feel terrible from the effects of the ablative therapy. They have severe irritation of the mucous membranes in the mouth, diarrhea, anorexia, fevers and chills, and lethargy. They are vulnerable to infections and bleeding, so everyone must scrub and wear masks, gloves, and gown when they enter the room."

David provided meticulous mouth care to Chip and urged him to get out of bed, shower, walk around the room, sit in the chair, and to try to eat. He teased and joked with Chip when Chip felt up to it, answered his questions and listened to his occasional expression of discouragement, checked on him frequently, and carefully monitored his pain medications.

Although Chip was suffering from the side effects of the radiation and chemotherapy, he appeared to be moving through the difficult process normally until day 14, when he developed severe chest pain. To everyone's surprise, an echocardiogram revealed congestive heart failure (CHF). It was not clear whether this was preexisting or had developed as a result of the regimen of the BMT. Chip received the news of the CHF with an effort at optimism, despite the fact that he was weak, nauseated, and now short of breath. He focused on his boys, reporting their latest school achievements.

The situation grew worse when Chip developed full-blown GVHD that caused red, raw blisters on his swollen feet and hands. Chip said he felt "rough" but added, "I'm trying to keep my spirits up." David recalled how, even when he was very ill, Chip joked about his now almost bald head, a side effect of the chemotherapy. David stepped up comfort measures, applying soothing ointment to Chip's blistered hands and feet, sitting with him whenever he could find time, just to help him get through some rough hours. Chip would ask how he was doing and David would answer him as honestly as he could. On one occasion Chip told David, "I know I'm not doing well. But I want you to know that

I want everything possible done for me. I can take suffering in the short term if I can live to see my boys grow up." David assured him that the team planned to support him fully and arranged for Chip to talk with the physicians, who also needed to hear his request.

Chip's cardiac problems increased, and the GVHD spread to his liver and gut, resulting in continuous diarrhea. Keeping him clean and dry required much of David's attention. Chip's care was complex. He needed a delicately orchestrated assortment of medications for the GVHD and CHF, with heavy doses of morphine to manage his pain. Because of the damage to his liver from the GVHD, he had trouble metabolizing his medications, and he grew confused and lethargic. Without a functioning immune system, he developed a fungus in his lungs and under his arms. Chip was now miserable and doing poorly. He asked that the boys not visit until he looked and felt better.

Frantic, Lois approached David and the physicians: "Promise me you will keep Chip alive. You've kept him going up until now. Don't stop." Sobbing, she concluded, "I simply cannot manage my life without him." The team assured Lois that they would do all they could.

Chip was sent for a biopsy to define what was happening in his lungs. When he was intubated for the biopsy, he began to bleed, and the bleeding was stopped only with great difficulty. After this episode, Chip was placed on a ventilator, unable to breathe on his own. At this point he was sent to the Medical Intensive Care Unit (MICU). Within days his liver and kidneys completely shut down. Renal dialysis was begun. The team was doing all they could to sustain Chip, but, despite the aggressive efforts, he was failing rapidly. Lois remained at the hospital for much of each day, visiting on the hour as the unit allowed. Aware that he was doing poorly, she urged the team to do all they could to save Chip.

No longer responsive, Chip was experiencing multisystem failure. He was swollen and no longer looked like himself. David visited him each day in the MICU. He explained, "I was upset. I wasn't sure we were doing the right thing trying to keep him alive. I wasn't sure whether we still might be able to save him. But we had promised him we would do what we could to sustain him and Lois was insisting we do everything possible for Chip." David decided to talk with the BMT team. "I wanted to know what others were thinking. I thought we could help each other know what to do. My concern was that we do what was best for Chip, and at that point, I didn't know what that was," he said.

The next morning during the daily team meeting, David questioned whether their interventions on Chip's behalf were now doing more harm than good. The discussion revolved around whether to continue to support Chip aggressively with the slim hope that he might pull through the crisis or to discontinue treatment. He now had three system failures—lungs, kidneys, and liver—and it was unlikely he could survive. The dilemma for the team was that despite Chip's limited chance of survival, they had promised to work aggressively to save him. After much discussion, the majority of the team concluded they should not "give up" on Chip yet. Justifying the decision, David said, "It was hard to turn away from the hope of saving Chip. No one wanted to do this prematurely, especially since we had promised Chip we would do all we could to save him. We were all very fond of Chip, and we were feeling sad over this turn of events. We were upset that he had developed such severe GVHD and we could not stop his decline." They decided to press on aggressively for three more days, then reassess the situation.

However, the next day Chip's brain waves were flat. David admitted, "Chip spared us the agony of having to decide to discontinue his life support when he became brain dead." Brain dead, there was nothing more to be done for him. Chip had died despite their determined efforts to save him. Now he needed to be taken off the ventilator.

When the MICU physician called Lois to report this, she protested, "I was just there. He was breathing. Don't stop his breathing machine." David understood her position. He said later, "Lois wanted a miracle. We now had to turn our attention to figuring out how we could help Lois." David, who among the team members knew Lois best, proposed they invite her to a meeting that afternoon and, as a team, try to help her see that Chip was dead and now must be taken off the machines.

They gathered that Saturday afternoon in a small conference room adjacent to the MICU—two BMT doctors, David, the MICU doctor, and Lois. David explained, "The meeting was tough. We were all deeply sad and disappointed. We had reached our limits with the technology. Lois could not accept those limits. For weeks she had witnessed many of the miracles of technology. Yet despite our best efforts, Chip had steadily declined. Now we couldn't fix Chip and she couldn't accept that reality." The MICU doctor explained to Lois that although Chip's chest was still moving because of the ventilator, he was legally and technically dead. The ventilator needed to be turned off.

Eventually Lois recognized that Chip must be taken off the ventilator. The question was when. Lois wanted to keep him on the ventilator until Monday so she and the boys could have time to say good-bye. The MICU physician, whose responsibility extended to the entire unit, wanted the ventilator to be turned off immediately. Arguing that Chip could no longer benefit from the MICU, he explained that his obligation to Chip had been met; his obligation now was to other patients waiting for a bed.

The BMT physicians and David felt some obligation to Lois but were not sure how to best meet her needs. Lois pleaded, "Please help me. I am not ready to turn off that machine. He is still breathing. It's like he is still with me. I need until Monday."

Hearing her plea, the MICU physician said, "Lois, we cannot tie a bed up that long. But I do want to help you."

David suggested a compromise. "Chip was a religious man," he said. "Tomorrow is Sunday, the Lord's day. How would it be if we turn off the ventilator after midnight tonight, on the Lord's day?"

David explained, "We had all played a part in getting to this point, and everyone wanted to help Lois. It seemed a reasonable compromise to me." The MICU physician hesitated and then said, "I guess we can go along with that."

Lois immediately got up and left the conference room. As she walked out she said to no one in particular, "It's only me and my boys now. Let me go be with the body." David observed, "With this statement you could see she was beginning to accept the inevitable."

Lois stayed with Chip late into the night. A family friend brought the boys by for a brief farewell. Lois and the boys were gone when the ventilator was turned off shortly after midnight.

"What was truly remarkable for me about this," said David, "was the courage of Chip, Lois, and the health care team. For all of us, when technology failed, we did not fail ourselves. We worked together until we reached an understanding about turning off the ventilator. Patients and families expect much from us, and they often get miracles. I learned that these miracles are of two sorts: life-saving miracles of technology and life-sustaining miracles of shared understanding."

Enacting Artful Nursing

Ethical nursing practice begins with a competent nurse whose knowledge and skills are sufficient to provide safe care. However, developing a sound knowledge base and mastering skills are only the first steps in building an ethical practice. David's story shows how his engagement with Chip and Lois brought understanding and compassion to a painfully complex and devastating experience. This discussion highlights three key nursing actions that demonstrate David's use of ethical knowledge as he cared for Chip and his family.

- Protecting vulnerable patients
- Understanding through dialogue
- Making ethical decisions

PROTECTING VULNERABLE PATIENTS

While nurses always seek to relieve suffering, the moral obligation to do so is particularly great when the patient's suffering is a direct result of the medical intervention (Gadow, 1988). Indeed, Gadow argues that at the point when efforts to cure overwhelm the patient to such an extent that the patient's suffering cannot be alleviated by care, the cure itself becomes morally questionable. David knew that the BMT caused extreme suffering. He explained his role as follows: "They suffer a lot. I try to relieve that suffering." David's struggle was to know at what point the team's efforts toward cure were no longer acceptable in terms of his commitment not to harm his patient.

David provided direct care to Chip, monitored Chip's pain medications, kept him clean and dry when he had diarrhea, and gently applied ointments to his blistered skin. David teased and joked with Chip, sat with him during painful periods, and checked on him frequently. He skillfully managed Chip's complex medication regimen as the GVHD progressed.

David's responses were directed in part by Chip's values. He knew that Chip appreciated learning, family, and religious beliefs. David taught him about the BMT, kept Chip informed about his physical status, asked about the boys, and talked with Chip about religion. When Chip told him he wanted to be treated aggressively, even if he had to "suffer in the short run," David arranged for Chip to talk with the physicians about this request and then joined the team's efforts toward that goal.

David's ethical struggle began when Chip went to the MICU. He began to question whether the treatment was causing Chip greater burden than benefit. Chip was unresponsive, and his body was deteriorating rapidly. He was so swollen that he no longer looked like himself. Chip's vulnerability was great; he had reached the point when he could no longer speak for himself. Chip had asked for aggressive treatment, but now further treatment appeared futile.

David's uncertainty turned on whether it was a violation of Chip's need to die to continue aggressive treatment. David struggled to know how to protect Chip from possible futile treatment while honoring his wish for aggressive intervention. David acknowledged, "I was upset. I wasn't sure we were doing the right thing." Propelled by this struggle, David met with the BMT treatment team and asked the question, Are we overtreating?

UNDERSTANDING THROUGH DIALOGUE

Ethical dilemmas involve differences in perspectives and values, not differences in facts. Hence, a feature of ethical practice is the ability to recognize and respect perspectives and values other than your own. Propelled by his growing uncertainty, David initiated a conversation with the BMT treatment team. His intention in talking with the team was significant: he did not argue for his perspective; rather he sought understanding. He said, "I wanted to find out what others were thinking. I thought we could help each other know what to do." This intention to understand other perspectives set the stage for the dialogue that followed. As team members talked, David learned that some questioned continued aggressive treatment while others felt they should press on. As is often the case when perspectives differ, a compromise was reached wherein the aggressive measures were to continue and be reassessed in three days.

The Saturday meeting with Lois also highlights the centrality of dialogue in seeking understanding. The focus was no longer on Chip but on Lois's request that Chip be maintained on the ventilator until Monday. Various perspectives were represented, each arising from different roles and experiences with Chip and Lois. David and the BMT physicians knew Chip and Lois. They had provided Chip's treatment and care. They had talked with him. They knew how much he loved his family, and they had witnessed his optimism and courage in the face of his declining physical status. They had promised to support him aggressively. They had watched as Lois kept vigil at Chip's bedside. From this perspective, they felt an obligation to consider Lois's request. "We couldn't just abandon Lois now that Chip was dead," David explained.

In contrast, the MICU physician had only seen Chip after he was intubated and unresponsive. He had not talked with Chip and he did not know him. His contact with Lois had been limited to a daily report on Chip's medical condition that he gave her each morning when he made his rounds. Aware that the BMT doctors were also in contact with Lois, he had limited his involvement to managing Chip's care in consultation with the BMT physicians. With little personal knowledge of Chip or Lois, he focused on the fact that Chip could no longer benefit from the MICU and other patients needed the bed.

Finally, Lois' perspective grew out of her intimate knowledge of and love for her husband Chip. She pleaded, "Please help me. I am not ready to let him go."

In this situation, no one perspective was truer than others; all could be justified ethically. Sharing the perspectives contributed to understanding among the participants. As Lois pleaded for more time with Chip while he was still on the ventilator, the MICU physician began to understand her perspective. "I want to help you," he said to Lois. Further, David's understanding now included a recognition of the MICU physician's need to make Chip's bed available to other patients. David's proposed compromise and its acceptance by the MICU physician arose from these expanded perspectives.

David's compromise blended compassion with the couple's religious values—the ventilator would be turned off on the Lord's day. Lois was given eight hours to say good-bye to her husband. This compromise reflected several aspects of the ethic of care. First, it reflected an individualized response to Lois that defied the usual medical procedure of immediately taking a brain dead patient off the ventilator. The compromise grew out of the BMT team's involvement with Lois. Because they were involved, the team knew what Lois wanted and they wanted to try to meet her needs. To ignore Lois would have been a violation of their relationship with her. The value of honoring relationships extended to all team members as they sought to understand each other rather than to force a particular perspective upon the group. Finally, the compromise was designed to meet the needs of everyone involved: Lois would have more time with Chip; the BMT team could honor their commitment to Lois; and the MICU physician would have a free bed in eight hours, a time frame he could accept.

MAKING ETHICAL DECISIONS

Four factors must be considered when making ethical decisions in health care: medical indications, patient preferences, quality of life, and contextual features (Jonsen, Siegler, & Winslade, 1998). No one factor exists in isolation from the others, although some may carry more weight in making treatment decisions than others, depending upon the situation. In David's story, medical indications and patient preferences were dominant themes in the team's discussions of Chip's treatment.

Medical indications include the patient's medical history, diagnosis, symptoms, prognosis, and treatment goals. Based on the principle of beneficence, the questions are always, How can the patient be benefited by medical and nursing care? and How can harm be avoided? (Jonsen et al., 1998, p. 13). Lack of clarity about Chip's prognosis and the best way to honor the principle of beneficence led to David's initial ethical distress and remained a focus of concern for the team until Chip was brain dead.

The influence of patient preferences in health care decisions is based on the principle of autonomy, which ensures that the "patient's right to choose [is] . . . respected to the extent possible in ethics and law" (Jonsen et al., 1998, p. 13). Both Chip's and Lois's preferences were well known and played key roles in treatment decisions. Indeed, the promise made to Chip to work aggressively on his behalf was a primary justification by the BMT team in their continued efforts to save Chip.

Perceptions of quality of life are directly tied to patient preferences since it is the patient's notion of quality of life that guides decision making. While the goal of treatment is to regain or maintain quality of life, Chip's experience shows that this is not always possible. If patients are to make informed treatment decisions, they need a truthful assessment of the impact of medical treatment upon quality of life. Chip was kept apprised of his physical situation until he reached a point where he could no longer participate in decisions. However, he had left a verbal advance directive about his notion of quality of life: he was willing to "suffer in the short run" to survive. The team followed his directive until he became brain dead.

Finally, contextual features include the effects of decisions on family and finances. Social concerns like the just allocation of scarce resources or other professional responsibilities of the doctor or nurse, such as the MICU physician's obligation to free Chip's bed for other patients, are also relevant contextual features (Jonsen et al., 1998). In the final meeting with Lois, the MICU physician said there was nothing more he could do for Chip, and other patients now needed the bed. Thus, he brought in the principle of just allocation of scarce resources as well as his professional responsibilities to patients beyond Chip.

Challenges to Ethical Practice

There are many obstacles to ethical practice by nurses. One of the main hindrances to protecting vulnerable patients is the fact that nurses have competing obligations. They are obligated to the organization for which they work, the physician, and the patient. While their primary obligation is to the patient (ANA Code, 1997), nurses are often unable to meet patient needs because of organizational or physician pressures. For example, in managed care systems nurses (and physicians) complain that patient needs are sometimes overlooked in an effort to reduce health care costs.

The professional values of nursing mandate that the nurse be mindful of patient needs, especially when efforts to meet these needs are constrained by organizational values. This is not easy, and there are times when patient needs simply cannot be met because of these constraints. For example, your patient may need an additional day in the hospital before discharge to regain more stamina, but the mandates of either hospital-imposed diagnosis related groups (DRGs) or the patient's insurance dictate an early discharge. While you can make a plea on behalf of your patient, you alone cannot change the system. You can, however, look for allies to support patient need–based decisions including other nurses and physicians. The critical factor is to never lose sight of the patient as the focus, even when your response to patient needs may be obstructed.

In hospitals, technology may also hinder efforts to alleviate patient vulnerability. While technology helps nurses work more efficiently, it may also decrease hands-on contact with the patient and impede nurse-patient interactions (Purnell, 1998), and it may be overused at the expense of the patient's well-being (McConnell, 1998). Further, the noise and demands of technology create a mighty obstacle to appreciating the quiet suffering and isolation of the patient who is hooked up to the machines (Locsin, 1998).

There are no easy solutions to the challenges of technology. First and foremost, you must see yourself as the bridge that spans the chasm (Gadow, 1988) between the vulnerable patient and the apparent invulnerability of the technology and practitioners surrounding the patient. By sharing the experience of the patient through remembering your own human vulnerability to illness and suffering, you can narrow the experiential gap between patient and nurse (Gadow, 1988).

There are also challenges to understanding through dialogue. In some settings and roles the nurse does not work with a collaborative team that welcomes different perspectives and engages in dialogue. In these situations, it is easy to feel victimized and lonely, but rarely is there a circumstance in which there is no one to talk with about ethical struggles. When a collaborative team is not available, even one colleague who will listen and talk is a good start toward creating a personal network for dealing with ethical struggles in practice. Further, most hospitals now have ethics committees who are willing to hear nurse concerns related to ethical matters.

Perhaps the greatest impediment to making ethical decisions is our own inexperience and insecurity. In most cases there is little clarity initially in ethical dilemmas. Recall how David said, "I didn't know what to do." In situations when we do not know what to do, the temptation to turn away is compelling, especially when we are busy nurses with many demands. However, willingness to engage in the struggle is the key to developing ethical nursing practice. You won't always get it right. Remember that you are developing an ethical practice, not a repertoire of "right answers." Further, you will not be able to take up every ethical challenge; some will be more compelling than others, and these are the struggles to engage in. The first requirement in building an ethical nursing practice is to be able to endure uncertainty and engage in a "sustained conversation whose goal might best be characterized as the discovery of what is right" (Bartholome, 1992, p. 10).

Summary

You may have experienced ethical conflict in your practice. If this is the case, you know that there are no easy solutions in such situations. The first step is to recognize a conflict. There also must be a willingness to engage in the conflict, that is, to participate in the ethical struggle. As you build your knowledge of ethics, clarify your personal values, develop your skills in supporting patient values, and continue to be socialized into the profession, you will develop skills in ethical comportment. Like all skills in nursing, facility in dealing with ethical issues improves with practice.

References

Bartholome, W. (1992). A revolution in understanding: How ethics has transformed health care decision making. *Quality Review Bulletin 1,* 6–11.

Beauchamp, T., & Childress, J. (1989). *Principles of biomedical ethics* (3rd ed.). New York: Oxford Press.

Code of Ethics for Nursing (Draft #7). (1997). American Nurses Association Center for Ethics and Human Rights. Washington, DC: ANA.

Davis, C.M. (1994). *Patient practitioner interaction.* Thorofare, NJ: Slack Publishers.

Davis, D.S. (1986). Nursing: An ethic of caring. *Humane Medicine, 1,* 19–25.

Gadow, S. (1988). Covenant without cure: Letting go and holding on in chronic illness. In J. Watson & M. Ray (Eds.), *The ethics of care and the ethics of cure* (pp. 5–14). New York: National League for Nurses.

Gilligan, C. (1982). *In a different voice.* Cambridge, MA: Harvard University Press.

Huggins, E.A., & Scalzi, C.G. (1988). Limitations and alternatives: Ethical practice theory in nursing. *Advances in Nursing Science, 10,* 43–47.

Jonsen, A.R., Siegler, M., & Winslade, W.J. (1998). *Clinical ethics* (4th ed.). New York: McGraw Hill.

Locsin, R.C. (1998). Technologic competence as caring in critical care nursing. *Holistic Nursing Practice, 12,* 50–56.

McConnell, E.A. (1998). The coalescence of technology and humanism in nursing practice: It doesn't just happen and it doesn't come easily. *Holistic Nursing Practice, 12,* 23–30.

Nursing's social policy statement. (1995). Washington, DC: American Nurses' Association.

Purnell, M.J. (1998). Who really makes the bed? Uncovering technologic dissonance in nursing. *Holistic Nursing Practice, 12,* 23–30.

Yeo, M., & Moorhouse, A. (1996). *Nursing ethics* (2nd ed.). Ontario, Canada: Broadview Press.

APPLICATION

....

ACTIVITY I
Group Discussion: Analysis of the Story

1. In David's story Lois approached him and the team with the plea, "Promise me you will keep Chip alive. You've kept him going up until now. Don't stop. I simply cannot manage my life without him." At this point the text states, "The team assured Lois that they would do all they could." It could be argued that the team and David failed Lois by not addressing her fears. How might they have addressed Lois's emotional needs? What could they have said to Lois? Do you think it would have made a difference in the outcome of the story if David or another nurse had taken the time to listen to her concerns? What reasons can you give for your responses.

2. At the point when Chip was experiencing multisystem failure, David questioned the team about whether the interventions on Chip's behalf were doing more harm than good. As a member of the team, what would your position have been and why?

3. After Chip died, the team met with Lois, who wanted to keep Chip on the ventilator over the weekend so she and the boys could say good-bye. How would you have responded to Lois's request? How would you justify your response?

4. Discuss the role of technology in this story. What are the benefits and burdens of health care technology as they are evidenced in this story? How did technology complicate Lois's understanding of what the team could do for Chip? How did technology complicate Chip's death?

ACTIVITY II
Case Analysis and Group Discussion:
Meeting Competing Needs

You are a nurse working in the MICU where Chip is a patient. For the last five days, you have been working with Mrs. Rand, a 58-year-old woman who was admitted with sepsis, an often fatal condition resulting from overwhelming infection. You have just weaned Mrs. Rand from the ventilator. She has been breathing on her own for less than 12 hours. She is still extremely ill and has severe anxiety from the trauma of her illness experience.

In report you learn that a new patient, Mr. Johns, is being transferred from a regional hospital and will be arriving in the MICU around 6 PM. There are no empty beds on the unit. The decision has been made to transfer your patient, Mrs. Rand, to a medical floor since she is the only patient on the unit who is not on a ventilator. You protest, citing Mrs. Rand's tenuous ability to breathe on her own and her anxiety.

"Why not transfer Chip?" you suggest. "He really should not be here at all. He has had no brain function."

In response, the unit supervisor describes the outcome of the patient conference held earlier that afternoon between David, the BMT and MICU physicians, and Lois. "Chip must remain on the MICU until just after midnight tonight," you are told. "There is no negotiation around this decision. The patient conference was difficult, his wife is extremely upset, and we cannot overrule their conclusion. I am very sorry. There really is nothing else to discuss," the supervisor concludes.

To make matters more complex, there are no other available ICU beds in the hospital at this time.

You are angry and upset. You cannot understand this decision. "Why should someone who cannot benefit from our services take a bed when my patient, who can benefit from our care, needs it?" you ask. "It does not seem fair to me," you protest.

BRIEF COMMENTARY

This is an ethical dilemma related to the fair distribution of scarce resources. It is not uncommon for nurses to have to decide similar resource issues, such as how to distribute one's time among ill patients with competing needs. It is important to assess these situations based upon patient need and expected outcome or benefit, without discrimination against any patient based on age, gender, race, or ability to pay.

Lois (as an extension of Chip, who is the identified patient), Mrs. Rand, and Mr. Johns all need to claim a MICU bed. Using the following questions as a guide, discuss this scenario. Be sure to keep in mind the ethical principles of justice and beneficence, the three ethical theories outlined in this chapter, and David's model of dialogue that seeks to understand the perspective of the other.

DISCUSSION QUESTIONS

1. Discuss the tension between the competing needs of the three patients—Lois (as an extension of Chip), Mrs. Rand, and Mr. Johns. Two patients (Lois and Mrs. Rand) are already in the system. Does this give their needs priority? What factors would you consider in deciding whose needs are greatest?

2. Given the expected arrival of Mr. Johns, should Lois's needs be reconsidered? If so, how would you approach reopening this discussion?

3. Do the MICU nurses have any moral or ethical obligation to Lois or Mr. Johns since they do not really know them and have not worked with them?

4. Discuss how the expected outcomes or benefits for Lois, Mrs. Rand, and Mr. Johns might influence your position. Who stands to benefit most from being in the MICU? Be sure to include a consideration of benefits beyond medical outcome. Is it appropriate in a MICU to consider factors beyond medical ones?

5. Recall the discussions in the patient care conference with Lois and the discussions in the nursing report. Explore any distinctions in the way the key players talked among themselves. What factors might have influenced these distinctions?

ACTIVITY III
Group Discussion: Resolving Ethical Dilemmas

Consider David's dilemma in regard to his concern that the team was overtreating Chip.

1. Describe his conflict.

2. What was at stake for Chip? For Lois? For David? For the BMT team?

3. Think about what you would have done had you been David. Use the four factors to be considered in making ethical decisions as your guide.

4. Justify your answer using the ethical knowledge described in this chapter.

ACTIVITY IV
Self-Reflection: Identifying Personal
and Professional Values

The following exercise in self-reflection is designed to help you identify your own values and the values of nursing that you support. Write your responses to each of the following questions.

1. Describe the values that were primary in your family.

2. Who declared these as values? What was the source of these values—parental authority, the Torah, the Bible, etc.?

3. How did you feel about these values? Were you largely compliant or did you defy the values?

4. Which of these values do you now hold?

5. Which have you discarded?

6. What values have replaced the family values you discarded?

7. On the basis of your current knowledge of nursing, what are the primary values of nursing?

8. Compare the values of nursing with your personal values.

ACTIVITY V
Self-Reflection: Thinking About Ethical Dilemmas

1. Describe an ethical dilemma that you have faced.

2. How did you feel?

3. If you were in the same situation again, would you make the same decision? If yes, why? If no, why not?

4. What did you learn about ethical decision making from this experience?

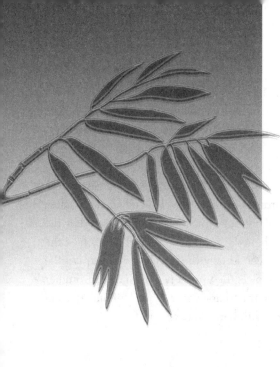

SECTION II

THE ART OF NURSING

....

The second section of this book looks at six concepts that you will need to understand in order to practice the art of nursing. These concepts are not the only concepts that are important to the art of nursing; however, they are central to artful nursing practice and frequently are used in discussions about the art of nursing.

The concepts depicted here overlap and are often simultaneously at play in patient care. Thus you can find evidence of each concept in every nurse story. However, each chapter in this section highlights only one concept because the concepts are initially best understood by highlighting one concept at a time.

Chapter 4 focuses on the central value of care. Elizabeth's care of her patient Leah depicts the complexity and skill required in artful nursing and the challenges to nurses who often feel impotent in the face of patient's enormous grief over dying. In Chapter 5, Jana portrays the art of advocating for a patient, Margaret, whose request to be kept alive until her grandchild was born presented multiple challenges. Chapter 6 looks at the story of Nancy, whose courage and commitment show how advocacy for populations can make an extraordinary impact upon the lives of many individuals. In Chapter 7, Gwyn's story demonstrates how the nurse respects and honors the patient's spiritual experience, regardless of whether the patient is facing the agony of loss or a peaceful acceptance of death.

Compassion is illustrated in Chapter 8 by Mark, a psychiatric nurse whose response to a patient with schizophrenia illustrates the challenging and healing nature of compassion. Chapter 9 is about nurse presence, demonstrated by the nurse Edith whose presence strengthened a young couple's ability to face the husband's aggressive and terminal cancer. Finally, the last chapter illustrates the art of caring for oneself. The story depicts the experience of Frances from her entry into nursing school, her growing frustration with the work of nursing, and her eventual satisfying reconciliation with her role in the profession.

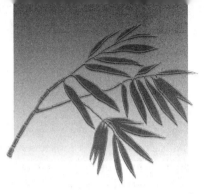

CHAPTER 4

Caring for Patients

Introduction

Caring has long been associated with the practice of nursing. Indeed, many students choose nursing as a career because they want to take care of people. They are drawn to vulnerable persons by natural traits such as kindness or compassion and a wish to alleviate suffering. However, caring involves more than kindness; caring is a way of being that arises from recognition of the fundamental connection or interdependence among all persons (Newman, 1997; Younger, 1995). Recognition of this kinship with others is based on an understanding that nurses share the same fate, joys, and sorrows as patients (Younger, 1995). Care arises from the wish to relieve the loneliness and suffering of a fellow human being.

The caring nurse is first of all a competent nurse (Cooper & Powell, 1998; Halldorsdottir & Hamrin, 1997). Without knowledge and competence, compassion and care are powerless to help the patient. However, the wisdom needed for care extends beyond scientific knowledge and technical competence and includes knowledge of the patient, the self, and the encounter between the self and patient. This knowledge is acquired through experience and practice.

In a little book titled *On Caring*, Meyerhoff (1971) wrote, "To care for someone, I must know many things. I must know, for example, who the other is, what his powers and limitations are, what his needs are, and what is conducive to his growth; I must know how to respond to his needs and what my own powers and limitations are" (p. 13). In other words, to care for patients, the nurse must have both general and particular knowledge.

This chapter highlights four basic aspects of care:
- Care as transformative
- Caring encounters
- Forms of care
- Rewards of care

Care as Transformative

Care matters! Consider the bewildered mother whose infant in the Neonatal Intensive Care Unit (NICU) was covered by tubes and surrounded by monitors. When the nurse took the time to explain the meaning of the technology, the mother felt great relief. Or consider the dying young man whose despair was eased when the nurse checked on him through a particularly long and scary night and held him as he wept. Consider the frightened parents who visited their daughter for the first time after her heart transplant and were told by the nurse, "It's OK to touch her. Go ahead and take her hand. Talk to her. She can hear you."

The absence of care also matters. Upon returning to her physician to have the stitches removed after a mastectomy, the poet Audre Lorde (1980) was chastised by a nurse for not wearing a breast prosthesis. The nurse scolded, "We really like for you to wear something, at least when you come in [to the office]. Otherwise, it's bad for the morale of the office" (p. 59). Lorde wrote, "I could hardly believe my ears! I was too outraged to speak then, but this was to be only the first assault on my right to define and claim my own body" (p. 59). Consider as well Carole Schroeder's experience. Upon hearing contradictory reports from two doctors about her critically ill baby's condition, Schroeder (1998) turned to the nurse for clarification. "[The nurse] just looked away, mutely refusing to get involved," said Schroeder, leaving her in "misery and isolation" (p. 16).

Patients describe noncaring encounters as "acid-edged and memorable experiences" (Halldorsdottir, 1991, p. 41). They describe uncaring nurses as "cold, cold human beings, like computers" (Halldorsdottir, 1991, p. 43) who are incompetent and indifferent, making patients feel distrust, disconnection, uneasiness, and discouragement (Halldorsdottir & Hamrin, 1997). Uncaring nurses withhold emotional support and come to patients' rooms only to perform tasks (Wolf et al., 1998). Denying patients' feelings, responding with indifference to patients' concerns, failing to see if a pain medication has worked for the patient, or not checking on a patient unless you have a procedure to perform can turn a terrible situation into a worse one. Such actions violate the patient's integrity and dignity and are never justified. This does not mean that the nurse must always have pleasant and uplifting encounters with patients. That is not possible. However, it does mean that the nurse always avoids comments or behaviors that are destructive to a patient's fundamental comfort, integrity, and dignity.

The power of care to ease or to sharpen suffering lies in its transformative nature. Care cannot take away confusion, grief, or pain, but a response of care can transform the fear and pain of illness and suffering into a tolerable, shared experience. Supported by responses of care, the mother of the NICU baby could focus on her baby's progress, the young man's night of grief was not quite so lonely, and the parents of the transplant patient were able to reach out to their daughter. In contrast, for Lorde and Schroeder, the absence of caring made terrible circumstances worse, leaving Lorde speechless with outrage and Schroeder miserable and isolated.

Caring Encounters

Many authors consider caring to be the essence and ideal of nursing (Benner & Wurbel, 1989; Newman, 1997; Watson, 1985). Their claim is based on the view that caring attends to the totality of the patient's experience (Newman, 1997), enhances dignity and instills hope (Watson, 1985), and enables an emotional connection that relieves the loneliness of the sufferer (Younger, 1995). In a caring encounter, the nurse does not step back to observe the patient but is engaged in the patient's experience. The focus is on the whole patient—emotional, spiritual, and physical (Newman, 1997).

Personal knowledge of the patient is the key to effective caring. The nurse needs to know who the patient is *in his uniqueness* (Carmody, 1994). For example, does the patient have a will to get better? Is she devastated or challenged by illness? Does he want to participate in all decisions? Ideally the nurse knows the patient's physical condition, coping resources, responses to pain, and values in relation to illness and health. As described in Chapter 2, personal knowledge is gained by talking with or observing the patient or directly asking the family about the patient. In his account of his experience with cancer, Carmody (1994) concluded, "Patients have a lot to tell their doctors, their nurses, their therapists, as the best people in such categories know well" (p. 37).

Knowledge of patient needs determines the caring response. This response requires skilled action; it is not enough simply to feel caring. For example, knowledge that the patient is in terrible pain does not mean simply that the nurse feels bad for the patient. Rather, this knowledge directs the nurse to assess how much pain medicine is needed, decide how quickly to return to see if the medication is working, when to reassess the pain, and how frequently to give medication.

Because human needs cannot always be anticipated, caring encounters may be uncertain and complex. Recall in Chapter 3 nurse David, who cared for Chip when he had a bone marrow transplant. At the beginning, David did not know how Chip's experience would turn out. Further, as the experience unfolded he did not always know what Chip needed, particularly in regard to further aggressive treatment. In the face of this uncertainty it would have been easy to disengage. David, however, remained involved and active on Chip's behalf, even after Chip became brain dead.

Forms of Care

Virginia Henderson defined nursing care as doing "those things the patient would do unaided for himself if he had the necessary strength, will or knowledge" (1966, p. 15). Caring responses are as varied as patients' needs and nurses' imagination, resources, and skills. Caring ranges from sitting quietly with a patient to performing complex treatments with sensitivity to the patient's response.

Caring encounters between nurses and patients vary in their intensity, duration, and frequency. They are influenced by the diversity of human responses, the stress of illness, the work demands of nurses, and the strengths and limitations of both nurses and patients.

The human connection in nurse-patient encounters is highly satisfying to most nurses, who describe bonds with patients as the "very cornerstone of patient care" (Ramos, 1992, p. 504). However, it is not possible—or desirable—to become intensely involved with all patients. Explaining the NICU equipment to the confused mother and pointing out small examples of her baby's progress did not require intense involvement with her. It did require openness to a connection with the mother, receptivity to the feelings of the mother, and knowledge of how to address her feelings. In her study, Ramos (1992) found that only a third of 67 descriptions of nurse-patient relationships depicted an intense emotional bond between the nurse and patient. While the intensity of the nurse-patient encounter varies, it *is* desirable to maintain a caring attitude toward all patients, conveying interest in their emotional and physical well-being.

Caring encounters also vary in duration. Some are brief and stand alone—as when your eyes meet those of a patient you do not know and you convey compassion and understanding. Other caring encounters extend over sufficient time to establish a relationship with the patient. An engaged and sustained relationship between patient and nurse is the ideal context for caring, since within this relationship the nurse has ample opportunities to get to know the patient and her needs. However, today nurses rarely have time to develop long-term relationships with patients. It is therefore important to recognize that while relationships enhance possibilities for caring, caring encounters with patients are not dependent on relationships. Recall in Chapter 1 Ben's response to Mrs. Floyd's terror during her carotid bleed. Ben's caring reassurance, arising from his recognition of the patient's fear, did not require a relationship between Ben and Mrs. Floyd. Similarly, Eliese's protection of the rights of her Jehovah's Witness patient to refuse blood did not require a developed nurse-patient relationship.

Finally, the frequency of caring encounters varies. All nurses do not have caring encounters with all patients. Some nurses are rarely caring with patients. For example, a 1991 study conducted in a long-term care facility found that caring interactions between elderly residents and nurses were scarce (Aventuro, 1991). Further, some patients are mean spirited and difficult to care for. Despite this, caring encounters are widely available to the responsive nurse and are daily fare for many nurses. One aspect of caring is an ability to recognize and seize opportunities for caring encounters with patients.

Rewards of Care

Whatever the intensity, duration, or frequency of caring encounters, caring creates a bond that is good for patients and nurses alike. As is evident in the stories in this text, care plays a central role in humanizing and cushioning episodes of illness (Eagleton & Goldman, 1997). Patients describe care as promoting a positive mental attitude and improved coping, movement toward recovery, increased physical comfort, as well as feelings of reassurance, trust, acceptance, satisfaction, and gratitude (Sherwood, 1993). Caring encounters have also been described as supporting patient and nurse growth (Mayerhoff, 1971). In an account of her experience as the mother of a newborn with a life-threatening heart defect, Schroeder (1998) described how a nurse periodically sat with her. "Her words and presence began to fill some of the emptiness inside me," (p. 19) said Schroeder. Simply talking with the nurse helped Schroeder find some meaning in the horror of her baby's illness as she "began to see that perhaps this experience wasn't just meaningless destruction, torture and death: regardless of outcome, we were all growing in ways denied ordinary people" (p. 20).

The nurse also gains from caring encounters. "Patients and healers are sharing a joint venture, even a joint (somewhat macabre) adventure," wrote an oncology patient. He continued, "This sharing can make us free. I feel free to ask about any problem and express any emotion, positive or negative. They, I hope, feel free to speak truthfully, to be playful or somber as the moment dictates. . . . All of us are simply people. Our lives are short" (Carmody, 1994, p. 37). Perhaps the most satisfying aspect of caring for patients is that it leads both the nurse and patient out of their own isolation into a human connection (Younger, 1995). As a result, caring is immensely gratifying. Even though caring often requires an emotional identification with the patient and may involve grief and sadness for the nurse, expert nurses are continually drawn into caring relationships because they are enriching (Ramos, 1992). Caring encounters provide opportunities for nurses to develop skills like listening, understanding, recognizing patient needs, and distinguishing between different emotional responses in patients. As these skills develop, the desire to help others that initially drew many nurses to the profession is fulfilled. Further, as the nurse pays attention to and modifies his responses to patient behaviors and feelings, the involvement with another person provides opportunities for self-knowledge and personal growth.

The story that follows depicts a caring relationship that developed over a period of ten months between Elizabeth and her patient Leah. The story shows caring to be hard and demanding work. Elizabeth used her finely developed caring skills, built upon a broad base of general knowledge and clinical experience, to alleviate Leah's immeasurable grief. Elizabeth recalled how at one point, the patient said to her, "Thank God you are here. In times like this, everyone needs a good nurse." Elizabeth replied, "Yes, we nurses would agree with that."

Elizabeth's Story

"There is only one story for me," Elizabeth began, "and that is the story of Leah. All the rest pale in comparison."

Elizabeth worked as an oncology nurse with a team of physicians and nurses whose practice included diagnosis, treatment, and home health care. A seasoned nurse, she cared for a caseload of patients in the clinic and in their homes. Her role included teaching, administering chemotherapy, managing pain and symptoms, and generally trouble-shooting.

Leah, a filmmaker, was a fashionable woman in her early forties, striking with her fair skin and long black hair. The most notable thing about Leah, however, was her joy in parenting her much-loved son. Her husband's work required that he travel, and Leah had happily assumed the primary responsibility for their child.

Leah's child had just celebrated his third birthday when Leah discovered she was pregnant again. She had suffered three early miscarriages, and Leah and her husband were delighted when she sustained this pregnancy past the critical third month. Then, during a routine obstetric checkup, Leah pointed out a reddened area on her breast. When the antibiotics did not reduce the redness, her obstetrician referred her as an emergency to the oncology clinic where Elizabeth worked.

A biopsy of the site indicated that Leah had inflammatory breast cancer, a lethal form of cancer. Without immediate and aggressive treatment, the cancer would spread like wildfire. Immediately Leah had to terminate the much-desired pregnancy because the chemotherapy would certainly kill the baby.

Elizabeth had only seen a few cases of inflammatory breast disease. She was stunned to see Leah's breast. Only two weeks after her initial symptoms, the redness extended from her now-misshapen breast to her underarm and around her back. The physician explained that a bone marrow transplant (BMT), the only possibility of a cure, was the ultimate goal. Meanwhile, Leah would have chemotherapy, then a mastectomy, followed by more chemotherapy and radiation. When they had the disease under control, Leah would be ready for the BMT.

Leah was both optimistic and determined. In her mind she simply could not die; she had a son who needed her. When she heard the diagnosis, she showed the physician and Elizabeth a picture of her child and said, "I have to live. I have to live for my son. I don't care what I have to go through. You have to keep me alive." The team promised to work with determination on Leah's behalf. Elizabeth herself had a three-year-old daughter. Recalling Leah, she said, "I had often thought that, apart from my child dying, the worst emotional pain imaginable would be to die and leave my young daughter without a mother. Now I had a patient who was facing this threat. I was drawn to her and wanted deeply to help her."

Leah's body scans were negative, indicating there was no evidence of metastases. Breathing a sigh of relief, Leah began the chemotherapy. Elizabeth taught Leah about the changes she would experience from the chemotherapy including hair loss, poor appetite, nausea and vomiting, and a general feeling of malaise. She taught her how to protect herself from infection since her immune system would be compromised. She suggested she have her long hair cut and pick out a wig.

Leah came to the clinic every three weeks for treatment. From the beginning, she suffered from nausea, vomiting, and weight loss. Elizabeth helped Leah identify comfort foods she might enjoy and urged her to ask her friends to prepare these special dishes for her when they wanted to help. Even when friends began to furnish Leah's meals, she continued to throw everything up. At this point, Elizabeth began home visits to monitor Leah's weight loss, blood studies, and her hydration.

Elizabeth felt an easy kinship with Leah, a bright and enthusiastic woman whose creative imagination was balanced by a down-to-earth appreciation of simple pleasures. She was the consummate mother. She gave her son careful attention and delighted in his developing personality. As Elizabeth and Leah talked, they learned that their children had been born on the same day, though in different hospitals. Leah's son arrived two months early, earning him a bed in the NICU. Elizabeth's daughter was full term, but because of a botched delivery she also went to the NICU. Both women had endured the agony of having a critically ill newborn and had anxiously followed the baby's first year of development. Happily, both three-year-olds were normal. The two women decided that when Leah got well, they would celebrate the children's next birthday together with a huge party.

After several rounds of chemotherapy, Leah was ready for the mastectomy. The clinic where Elizabeth worked was part of a large university-based hospital. Therefore, when Leah asked Elizabeth to accompany her to the operating room (OR), Elizabeth was able to do so. The scene was eerie for Elizabeth who recalled her feelings: "It was like that scene in *Dead Man Walking*, the movie in which the nun walks with the condemned man to the room where he will die. I had this strange sense that we were walking together to some inevitable place. Even though I hoped this was a life-saving experience, I could not get that image from my mind."

Elizabeth left Leah in the OR. On her way back to the clinic, she kept thinking of her patient. "It was at this point," she recalled, "that I realized I was deeply connected to Leah and this was going to be painful for me, especially if Leah did not survive. I also realized that Leah was increasingly dependent on me to help her through this experience. Leah had become one of those patients who come along every once in a while and get under your skin in a good way, but also in a way that is hard. So, I made the commitment to myself to be there for the duration."

Elizabeth was not the only person who felt involved with Leah. Everyone who worked with her liked her. Elizabeth recalled, "Leah was a beautiful woman who embodied a strange mixture of optimism and deep grief. It was like she held herself in a circle of hope and light, and those caring for her were drawn into that circle. She was profoundly grateful for anything we were able to do for her. And yet at the center of her experience there was an intense sadness at the threat of leaving her young son. We all wanted to relieve that sadness, to comfort her, support her optimism, and sustain her hope."

Several weeks after the surgery, Leah resumed chemotherapy and began radiation. After what seemed an eternity, she was finally ready to be worked up for the hoped-for BMT. Scans were done to ensure there was no metastasis. To everyone's horror, despite the aggressive treatment the scans showed extensive metastases. Upon hearing the news from the radiologist, Leah came to Elizabeth's office sobbing, "It's everywhere. It's in my liver, my bones. It's even in my brain."

"The cancer was like a freight train that couldn't be stopped," Elizabeth recalled.

Leah's grief was inexpressible. Her deepest longing was to live for her son. At first she hoped to live until his college graduation, then high school, and then kindergarten. As she scaled back her expectations, her grief intensified. Yet despite the grief, Leah managed to have happy times with her son. On good days she would take him to the park or join him in his play. She took him to the library and read to him. When she could tolerate the smells, she would take him out to eat at his favorite fast food places.

Leah began to count heavily on Elizabeth, calling her with questions and looking forward to Elizabeth's home visits. During these visits, Leah would talk with Elizabeth about her fears and hopes, all of which focused on her son. Elizabeth recalled, "She would describe the latest outing with her son and then be overtaken by grief at the possibility of having to leave him. She didn't express her grief with many people. I think I provided the safety she needed to share her feelings without the threat of someone judging her or trying to make her hard feelings go away."

Leah's husband also counted on Elizabeth. Unable to deal with the possible loss of his wife, he became increasingly distant as Leah's situation grew worse. His travel picked up; Leah accepted this. It was hard, however, for Elizabeth to witness, because Leah needed his support. But Elizabeth soon recognized, "I had to let him be who he had to be. He loved her but could not be there for her. Yet his absence was a loss for Leah and for him."

Despite the metastases, Leah wanted to press on aggressively with more chemotherapy and radiation to her brain. Nothing helped. The freight train barreled ahead. There was little time to deal emotionally with the onslaught of the illness. Focused on Leah's deep grief, Elizabeth recalled, "It happened so quickly. She was always playing catch-up, trying to process the latest blow when another one came along. She would still be reeling from one thing when she had to deal with something else. It was a bereavement overload."

Eventually it became clear that the chemotherapy was killing Leah, who could not eat and whose immune system was drastically compromised. There was no choice but to stop the treatment and give Leah a rest. For the first time since she had begun treatment, Leah felt pretty good. She gave herself a birthday party, inviting several families, including Elizabeth's, to a potluck. The friends brought food, cake, and gifts for Leah, who also wrapped a gift for each of her friends. When she cut her cake, she told those gathered, "When I get well, I'm going to rent a villa in Tuscany and have everyone over as a thank you for what you are doing for me." There was no doubt in anyone's mind that if she lived, Leah would fulfill this promise.

Four days later a physician friend of Leah's gave a surprise party for her. It was a fine affair, by the best caterer in town, and included all her friends and many of the professionals caring for her, all dressed in their party best. Arriving after the guests had gathered, an unsuspecting Leah was met with shouts of "Surprise! Surprise." Laughing and crying she repeated, "Thank you. Thank you." While at the party, Elizabeth talked with the wife of Leah's radiologist, who confided, "My husband doesn't get involved with many patients. About once a year he has a patient whom he calls his 'connection' patient. He bonds with that patient. Leah is his connection patient. Now I understand what drew him to her. She is radiant in her courage and gratitude."

Leah's reprieve from feeling wretched was short-lived. Without chemotherapy, the cancer grew rapidly. Leah pressed on. Still unable to eat, she requested a nasogastric (NG) tube and bolus feedings in the hope that she could gain some weight and strength and resume treatment. Elizabeth wasn't sure it was worth the pain and discomfort for Leah to have an NG tube, but aware of Leah's longing to stay alive for her son, the team supported her request without question. After a painful and tedious effort, the NG tube was finally in place. Leah immediately vomited. Turning to Elizabeth, she asked, "What was I thinking when I asked for this?"

"You were thinking that you want to keep going, keep trying to get better so you can start treatment again. You can't eat and you wanted nourishment," Elizabeth reminded her patient.

"Yes, I remember. Thank you," Leah replied.

Leah was too weak to give herself the bolus feedings and her husband, continuing to fade out of the picture, could not help. Elizabeth stepped up her home visits and trained Leah's neighbors and friends to give the bolus. Despite the feedings, Leah continued to worsen. Her liver doubled in size, and within a few weeks she could not leave her bed.

Leah did not complain of physical pain despite bone metastases throughout her body. She never spoke about her own death. Her talk was always about leaving her child. Despite her efforts, Elizabeth felt that she could not begin to touch Leah's grief. Elizabeth recollected, "I did not know there could be such deep sadness. Never before had I had a patient who remained inconsolable. Perhaps other patients hid their grief. I do not know. It was very hard."

Once, in an effort to give comfort, Elizabeth said to her patient, "Maybe you'll be your son's guardian angel when you die."

"No," Leah came back, "I believe when I die I'm gone and that's it." Leah did not believe in an afterlife. There was no comfort for her there. When she died, it would be over.

Elizabeth felt impotent. "The only thing I could do, or anybody could do for her grief, was just be there and listen. I could not change it. There was nothing to say that did not sound cheap and stupid. I could not say, 'This is going to be all right' because it wasn't all right, none of it was all right. I couldn't say, 'Your baby will be fine,' because I didn't think he would be fine and she didn't either. There was nothing to say." And so without words, Elizabeth would hold Leah or gently give her a warm bath. Often as she held Leah, Elizabeth would feel her own sadness and be comforted by the thought, This is the best of what nurses do. This is why I became a nurse.

Elizabeth was soon making a home visit almost every day. Her nursing care now included providing comfort by keeping Leah's skin lubricated and her elimination under control, rubbing sore body parts, managing Leah's pain medication, and assessing her for physical changes including swelling, breath sounds, and changes in her liver. She helped make her room more comfortable by arranging to have a hospital bed and a TV and VCR brought in. With some caution, she recommended that hospice begin home visiting. Confined to bed and declining rapidly, Leah agreed to have the hospice nurse assist with her care. With Leah's permission, Elizabeth arranged for the rabbi to come and talk with Leah. Still, Leah's grief remained constant.

Reflecting on her role, Elizabeth declared, "I did all that was humanly possible for her and I took comfort in that. But the pain of leaving her child was so profound and intense that there was nothing I could do to relieve it. Yet I do believe my presence helped her. Presence can help when the pain is very deep. Presence can make things a little better."

As Leah's condition worsened, the hospice nurse made daily visits. Leah's sister, who had visited often during her illness, came to stay. Leah's son did not understand. Alternating between playing and clinging, he would crawl into bed with his mother but soon become restless and leave again. At Leah's request, equipment was gathered to make an audiotape for her son. Although it was a good idea, Leah could never bring herself to make the tape. She tried to talk to her son, to explain her dying. "Mommy's been real sick and now I have to leave. I'm going to die. Daddy will take care of you," she said. It was not the kind of connection she wanted. He was too young and didn't understand.

The hospice nurse who worked with Leah noted her restlessness. Concluding that it was not related to pain, the nurse called Elizabeth to ask, "Why is she upset? I don't think she is in pain but she seems upset. Help me understand. I don't know her well."

"She doesn't know how to leave her child. Her grief is profound," Elizabeth told the concerned nurse.

As Leah's death neared, Elizabeth was mostly relieved. She wanted this to end. Leah's death was inevitable, and Leah had suffered enough. Elizabeth reflected, "It was really tough. It was the suffering that was so hard, the desperation to stay alive and my total inability to stop this oncoming freight train. There were things I could do, but I could not affect the outcome. I wanted to shout, 'Can't we do something about this? Doesn't anyone have a trick up her sleeve?' Finally, I realized that, on the one hand, there was nothing to do. Yet on the other hand, there were still things that I could do."

Recognizing that her patient was close to death, Elizabeth spoke to Leah, helping her to die. "Don't worry that you didn't make the tape for your son," she said. "There are a lot of things you wanted to do that you didn't get a chance to do. It's all right. Your friends and family will make sure your son knows and remembers you. You have other videotapes, and your family has memories. It is OK. It is time. You need to go." Elizabeth explained, "She loved her son so much and hated to leave him without a mother. I felt she needed that last reassurance."

Within an hour of this reassurance, Leah died with her sister and husband at the bedside and her son asleep in the next room. Elizabeth returned to Leah's home. With deep sadness she noticed that Leah's face looked pained and far from peaceful. She took her hand and sat with her until the hospice nurse arrived. She recalled, "After she died some part of her stayed there for a little while and I could not leave her. And then there was a time when I realized her spirit was gone. However, at first, I knew that something wasn't gone yet and so I just sat quietly with her for a while."

Elizabeth and the hospice nurse worked together to bathe and dress Leah. The hospice nurse kept repeating, "Lord have mercy, Lord have mercy."

"It was as if she were trying to invoke some mercy on these pain-filled circumstances." Elizabeth explained.

Having cleaned and dressed Leah, Elizabeth called for her sister and husband to come and say good-bye. Leah's sister walked into the room. Startled, she asked Elizabeth, "How did you do that?"

"What?" Elizabeth inquired.

"How did you make her face look like that? She looks like an angel and she is smiling," Leah's sister exclaimed.

Turning to Leah, Elizabeth noted that the tortured look was indeed gone. "We didn't do anything," she said. "We didn't touch her face except to wipe it with a cloth. And yes, you are right, she is smiling."

Two years later, Elizabeth recalled the experience with her patient Leah: "It was like a drive-by shooting—quick, random, and obscene. There was no window of remission for her to deal with it and to adjust her dreams. It happened so quickly that she could not assimilate it. There was little to do but listen. I think my listening validated Leah's experience. The experience also validated for me what being a nurse really means. I learned that while I cannot necessarily change the outcome, I can ease the journey to the inevitable a little bit. When there is no cure and nothing to say, there are still things that I can do that make a difference."

Enacting Artful Nursing

Elizabeth's expert skills, receptivity to Leah, and willingness to be involved set the stage for an ideal enactment of nursing care. Her story highlights the enduring nature of care that sustains patients in the face of inexpressible grief and the failure of efforts at cure. Elizabeth's story illustrates three key nursing actions.

- The activities of care
- Knowledge and skills of care
- Care as connection

THE ACTIVITIES OF CARE

There is a vast difference between feelings of care and actions of care. It is easy to feel caring. Indeed, most health care professionals care about whether patients get well and feel sorry when they do not. However, it is hard to engage in caring behaviors. Even though Leah's husband loved her, he was not engaged in caring for her. He cared how things turned out for her, but because he lacked the skills of care and failed to become involved, his caring was limited.

In contrast, Elizabeth's care was hands-on, involved, active caring that required skill and effort. She rubbed her patient's aching body, bathed her, helped her manage her diarrhea and constipation, administered her bolus feedings, sustained her hope, listened to her grief, sat quietly with her or held her when there were no words of comfort. These activities of care took time, but they also required skill, an intentional focus on Leah's needs, and a desire to relieve Leah's suffering. In today's health care environment, where time is scarce, Elizabeth's focus on Leah provides an excellent example of the foundations of caring.

An expert nurse, Elizabeth's caring skills were built on theoretical and experiential knowledge, and she was at home with the work of care. Elizabeth also actively made the choice to care when she opened herself to involvement with Leah. From this posture of openness she found that, indeed, Leah had gotten "under her skin." She knew that caring for Leah could hurt, and she would at times feel sad or impotent in her efforts. She also knew that caring was the best of nursing. With all this in mind, Elizabeth made the commitment to be there for the duration of the experience.

KNOWLEDGE AND SKILLS OF CARE

Caring requires a solid base of knowledge and skills (Benner & Wurbel, 1989). First and foremost, Elizabeth was competent. She had skills in both assessment and intervention with cancer patients. She understood the treatment protocol and how to prepare Leah for treatment. She understood how to administer the chemotherapy and how to assess and manage its side effects. She comprehended the importance of assessing nutritional and elimination patterns, and she also knew how to intervene when problems arose. She could put down an NG tube, manage bolus feedings, and teach Leah's friends how to help. She knew how to assess for discomfort and pain and how to medicate. In short, Elizabeth knew what to look for, what to do, and how to do it. Armed with this knowledge, she assessed Leah's physical responses to the cancer and its treatment and intervened appropriately.

Elizabeth also understood the nature of caring. She acknowledged the contradictions of care when she embraced the fact that caring was "good and hard" at the same time. The openness to the patient's experience required in caring meant that Elizabeth would hurt when her patient hurt. It also made possible deep personal and professional satisfaction. Elizabeth knew that while her caring was focused on Leah, it also enriched her and brought her closer to the ideal of nursing. She would hold Leah without words and remember, This is the best of what nurses do. This is why I became a nurse. At the same time, It was very hard.

Elizabeth also knew that caring is a privilege not to be lightly passed up. This was evident in her observation that the lack of involvement constituted a loss for Leah's husband. Elizabeth pointed out the abiding nature of care when she noted that when there was "nothing left to do" to bring about a cure, there was still much she could do to care. She could not stop the progression of Leah's disease, but she could offer her quiet presence. She could not make Leah's grief go away, but she could ease the journey to the inevitable.

Elizabeth relied upon knowledge of herself to guide her caring. She recognized that her involvement with Leah was going to be painful. This was true for Elizabeth because, as she cared for Leah, she grew attached to her. Through her caring she recognized in Leah the suffering that, on some level, all humans share: she too was vulnerable to suffering. Their relationship was genuine, without pretense or false efforts. She needed to comfort Leah, and Leah did not need to hide her grief. Leah felt fully her inexpressible grief, without interference from a nurse who could not bear witness to her pain. Neither denied the tragedy in this situation, and Elizabeth provided the safety Leah needed to express her deep sadness without the threat of someone's judging her or trying to make her hard feelings go away.

Elizabeth's competence and self-knowledge were the cornerstone for her nursing care, but she also needed knowledge of Leah to personalize her care. She came to know Leah as Leah understood herself. First and foremost, Leah was a mother. Noting that Leah's grief about leaving her son was more important than her own physical pain and approaching death, she could appreciate Leah's deep, profound, and intense pain and avoid the temptation to trivialize her grief with false reassurance. She knew what Leah needed physically to be comfortable, noting how a warm bath was comforting and where to rub her body to provide pain relief. She learned what Leah liked to eat. Elizabeth knew details like Leah's wish to make a tape for her son. When she realized that Leah, near death, could not fulfill that wish, she helped to release her from the effort when she said, "It is all right. Your friends and family will make sure your son knows and remembers you . . . you need to go."

CARE AS CONNECTION

Elizabeth's initial connection with Leah was natural and easy. She liked Leah and, like other health care providers, was drawn to Leah by attractive qualities like courage, determination, optimism, and hope. Further, Leah was facing what Elizabeth recognized as "the worst emotional pain imaginable," and Elizabeth's wish to help her through the experience also drew her to Leah.

The connection with Leah moved to a new level of intensity for Elizabeth as she accompanied her patient to the OR for her mastectomy. They were "walking together to some inevitable place," even though Elizabeth did not know how this would turn out. Their connection depended upon an attitude of openness on the part of both women. Each was receptive to the other. There is not always an easy rapport between the nurse and patient. However, care depends not on easy rapport but on the recognition that in terms of human experiences, we are all connected (Younger, 1995). Recognizing this deep human connection, Elizabeth reached out to Leah.

Within their connection, Elizabeth recognized that her presence was one means of relieving the *isolation* of Leah's unspeakable grief and suffering. She could not take away Leah's grief, but Elizabeth believed that "presence can help when the pain is very deep. Presence can make things a little better."

Younger (1995) describes presence as "the most demanding and deeply human aspect of caring. . . . In the deepest sense, caring for the other is extending a human and humane presence to a fellow being" (p. 68). Elizabeth's presence took the form of listening as Leah talked, holding her, and quietly sitting with her. Their connection extended beyond Leah's death when Elizabeth, recognizing Leah's presence in the room after she had died, sat quietly holding her hand until "her spirit was gone."

In a little book called *Traveling Mercies,* Lamott (1999) describes her response to her friends whose child had recently been diagnosed with cystic fibrosis. She wrote, "Sometimes we let them resist finding any meaning or solace in anything that had to do with their daughter's diagnosis, and this was one of the hardest things to do—to stop trying to make things come out better than they were. We let them spew when they needed to; we offered the gift of no comfort when there being no comfort was where they had landed" (p. 152). Elizabeth's story depicts the gift of caring without the trappings of making everything right.

Challenges to Caring for Patients

Elizabeth's story of care is an ideal example of caring. Elizabeth's role allowed her to establish an ongoing relationship and follow Leah in the clinic and in her home; the natural affinity between the women initially made caring easier, and the openness of both made possible a deep connection. Despite relative silence about the failures of care in the nursing literature (Halldorsdottir & Hamrin, 1997), the ideals of caring are often not actualized in nursing. There are multiple constraints to caring that are both internal and external to the nurse.

Externally, there are many constraints to the activities of caring. Nurses are expected to be caring in a system that is driven by economics, not care. Economic compensation for caring is difficult because of the invisibility of caring, which occurs in the privacy of the nurse-patient encounter (Radsma, 1994). Furthermore, nurses are not specifically held accountable for caring behaviors.

Unfortunately, nurses contribute to the devaluing of caring by their inability or unwillingness to speak up about their caring work, knowledge, and skills. It is difficult to expect organizations driven by economics to value care if nurses themselves do not talk about their caring. Nurses may minimize their care by "comments such as 'don't worry about it; it wasn't much . . .' or 'it was the least I could do. . . .' [Such comments] reveal a subtle form of self-depre-cation by nurses toward the expertise required to carry out the work of nursing care" (Radsma, 1994, p. 447).

With downsizing, fewer nurses are caring for more and sicker patients and nurses are doing more with less, a situation that taxes nurses to their limits (Miller, 1995). Nurses are now expected to coordinate many aspects of patient care while working with greater workloads and sicker patients. It is little won-der that caring is often difficult, given the competing demands on the nurse. However, receptivity to the patient is key to every caring practice. It does not take any extra time to maintain an attitude of kindness, courtesy, gentleness, and receptivity to the patient. While it does take time to listen to patients, you will find that as you master technical skills, you will be able to do the tasks of nursing while attending to the patient so that you can get to know the patient as you are doing an assessment or treatment.

It is important to remember that caring is an attitude, a way of being with a patient, and a set of skills that can be learned and developed, and that require nurturing and attention. Tell your stories of caring. Point out to others how car-ing matters to patients and nurses. Confront those who diminish the importance of caring by speaking up on behalf of care and urging colleagues to "let caring 'civilize' the not-so-civilized current healthcare industry [by remembering] that without caring we would be like every other business" (Miller, 1995, p. 32).

There are also internal constraints to the activities of care. Some nurses do not know how to protect themselves from feeling overwhelmed by the patient's experience. Nurses have described being swallowed up by patient suffering and unable to step away from the patient's experience to avoid feeling devastated themselves (Ramos, 1992, p. 501). Other nurses are uncaring or they lack com-passion and respect for patients, resulting in distancing behavior. Their indif-ference, reflected in a cold and sterile approach, is manifested by not listening to patients, keeping patients waiting for medication, giving assistance with no explanation, or being sarcastic, accusing, or careless (Halldorsdottir & Hamrin, 1997).

In some situations, nurse behaviors may be well intentioned and appear caring though in actuality they distance the nurse from the patient and protect the nurse from feeling anything for the patient. For example, excessive or un-realistic optimism may shield the nurse (and patient) from the difficulty of fac-ing feelings of discouragement. Other distancing behaviors include offering false reassurances that may sound comforting but effectively silence anxious patients such as "It will be OK" or "Now don't you worry." Efforts to control or dominate the decision making, ostensibly in an effort to relieve the patient of this burden, may diminish the patient's self-determination while relieving the nurse of engaging in shared decision making.

Acting like a "supernurse" is another way to distance oneself. Schroeder described such a nurse thus: "Spinning around the cubical, cleaning, dusting, and rearranging supplies, she handled Morgan [the baby] briskly, oblivious to my or to Morgan's distress" (1998, p. 15). Similarly, working with the technology rather than the patient can distract the nurse from caring involvement. Finally, feeling victimized by the demands of work shuts the nurse down to caring encounters. Hiding behind loud sighs and hurried distracted behavior, the victimized nurse signals that there is no time to listen to patient concerns and eliminates the possibility of genuine encounters with patients.

Many of these behaviors are forms of self-deception, and they are confusing to nurses and patients alike. Rather than engage in self-deception, it is much more useful to acknowledge your limitations in caring for others while remaining receptive to caring connections. It is normal to feel uncaring at times. Sometimes the nurse is burned out or overextended; sometimes difficult patients provoke uncaring feelings. It is particularly difficult to be caring toward patients who direct their anger at the nurse. In the face of patient anger, many nurses "disconnect" because patient anger is perceived as a threat to the nurse's sense of adequacy (Smith & Hart, 1994).

Interestingly, Smith and Hart's 1994 study showed that as nurses gained experience, they were able to minimize that response to patient anger by not taking the anger personally and recognizing anger as a normal part of some illness experiences. Experienced nurses were also able to recognize their own anger toward the patient and deal with this by taking a deep breath, slowly counting, or leaving the room for a few minutes until they were calm. It is never easy to be the object of a patient's anger, but nurses report that with experience, effective responses to patient anger can be developed, particularly if the nurse works in a supportive environment (Smith & Hart, 1994).

Given all these obstacles to caring, what is a good nurse to do? As you enter the profession, it is important to recognize that while caring is the ideal of nursing and a source of professional satisfaction, there are limits to caring. You cannot have an intense caring relationship with all your patients. You will not like all your patients. You will not even want to be caring on some days. However, being a nurse entails certain fundamental obligations, regardless of the demands of the work setting or your personal inclinations. First and foremost, you must be competent and always avoid uncaring responses to patients, regardless of how you feel. This does not mean that you do not protect yourself from abusive patients or systems. It does mean that, bound by the moral obligations of the profession, you rise above personal inclinations to ignore the needs of unlikable, angry, or demanding patients and address their needs. Paradoxically, openness to connections with patients, regardless of their personal characteristics, is often the key to diminishing the constraints presented by angry patients to caring.

Summary

The power of care to transform difficult, even tragic situations into shared human experiences that are tolerable and, in some cases, good, makes caring essential to the well-being of patients and nurses alike. Caring encounters involve a choice to become involved, a focus on patient needs, and active and individualized responses to those needs. While caring encounters vary in their intensity, duration, and frequency, they are all characterized by recognition of a common humanity that binds nurses and patients together. And they all involve an effort to reach out to a fellow sufferer. Development of your caring skills, including scientific and technological competence, is the key to artful nursing. With these skills in place, there will be patients whose stories will touch you and you will become involved with them. Soon you will have stories to tell just like the stories you are reading in this text.

References

Aventuro, B.A. (1991). The meaning of care to geriatric persons living in a long term care institution. *Dissertation Abstracts International, 52,* 2988B.

Benner, P., & Wurbel, J. (1989). *The primacy of caring.* Menlo Park, CA: Addison-Wesley.

Carmody, J. (1994). Bad care, good care, and spiritual preservation. *Second opinion, 20*(1), 35–39.

Cooper, M.C., & Powell, E. (1998). Technology and care in a bone marrow transplant unit: Creating and assuaging vulnerability. *Holistic Nursing Practice, 12*(4), 57–68.

Eagleton, B.B., & Goldman, L. (1997). The quality connection: Satisfaction of patients and their families. *Critical Care Nurse, 17*(6), 76–180, 100.

Halldorsdottir, S. (1991). Five basic modes of being with another. In D.A. Gaut & M.M. Leininger (Eds.), *Caring: The compassionate healer* (pp. 37–49). New York, NY: National League for Nursing.

Halldorsdottir, S., & Hamrin, E. (1997). Caring and uncaring encounters within nursing and health care from the cancer patient's perspective. *Cancer Nursing, 20,* 120–128.

Henderson, V. (1966). *The nature of nursing.* New York, NY: Macmillan.

Lamott, A. (1999). *Traveling mercies.* New York, NY: Pantheon Books.

Lorde, A. (1980). *The cancer journals.* San Francisco, CA: Spinsters/Aunt Lute Press.

Mayerhoff, M. (1971). *On caring.* New York, NY: Harper and Row.

Miller, K.L. (1995). Keeping the care in nursing care: Our biggest challenge. *Journal of Nursing Administration, 25*(11), 29–32.

Newman, M.A. (1997). Experiencing the whole. *Advances in Nursing Science, 20*(1), 34–39.

Radsma, J. (1994). Caring and nursing: A dilemma. *Journal of Advanced Nursing, 10,* 444–449.

Ramos, M.C. (1992). The nurse-patient relationship: Theme and variations. *Journal of Advanced Nursing, 17,* 496–506.

Schroeder, C. (1998). So this is what it's like: Struggling to survive in pediatric intensive care. *Advances in Nursing Science, 20*(4), 13–22.

Sherwood, G. (1993). A qualitative analysis of patient responses to caring: A moral and economic imperative. In D.A. Gaut (Ed.), *A global agenda for caring* (pp. 243–255). New York, NY: National League of Nursing Press.

Smith, M.E., & Hart, G. (1994). Nurses' responses to patient anger: From disconnecting to connecting. *Journal of Advanced Nursing, 10,* 643–651.

Watson, J. (1985). *Nursing: Human science and human care.* Norwalk, CT: Appleton-Century-Crofts.

Wolf, Z.R., Colahan, M., Costello, A., Warwick, F., Ambrose, M.S., & Giardino, E.R. (1998). Relationship between nurse caring and patient satisfaction. *MEDSURG Nursing, 7*(2), 99–105.

Younger, J.B. (1995). The alienation of the sufferer. *Advances in Nursing Science, 17*(4), 53–72.

APPLICATION

....

ACTIVITY I
Group Discussion: Analysis of the Story

1. Leah's grief was deeply felt and she was inconsolable about having to leave her young child. Discuss Elizabeth's response to Leah's deep grief. What did she do? What did she choose *not* to do? How would you have responded to Leah's sadness?

2. Discuss the features of grief such as Leah's that make it difficult for the nurse to be "present" with the patient. Why was it so painful for Elizabeth to stay connected to Leah? What feelings arise in a nurse who cares for a patient whose emotional suffering cannot be relieved?

3. How would you have responded to Leah's husband when he began to distance himself from his dying wife? What else could Elizabeth have done? How could the nurse, or perhaps the physician, have addressed Leah's husband's needs?

4. Caring for Leah was hard work. What do you think enabled Elizabeth to maintain her commitment to and engagement with Leah?

ACTIVITY II
Group Discussion: Activities of Caring

Review Elizabeth's story.

1. Identify the *activities* of care like touch, listening, pain management, etc., that are in Elizabeth's story.

2. Discuss the caring activities (identified in Question 1) that require an extensive time commitment by the nurse.

3. List the caring activities (identified in Question 1) that do not require an extensive time commitment by the nurse.

4. Discuss the claim that caring requires so much time that nurses can no longer care in today's hectic health care system. Do you believe this to be true? If so, describe how the profession of nursing, without caring, would differ from any economically driven enterprise.

ACTIVITY III
Group Discussion: The Experience of Caring

1. Discuss how Leah's experience would have differed had Elizabeth remained aloof and indifferent to Leah. Would her medical care have been any different? What about her physical and emotional care? Be specific in your descriptions of what would have been different for Leah.

2. How would Elizabeth's experience have been different if she had remained aloof and indifferent to Leah? Would she have remembered Leah's story? Would she have hurt in the ways she did? Would it have been easier or more difficult to remain distant? Be specific about what would have been different for Elizabeth.

3. Discuss how caring for patients affects the nurse *personally*.

4. Describe verbal and nonverbal behaviors that nurses display expressing genuine presence, respect, understanding, and caring.

5. Describe verbal and nonverbal behaviors that nurses display expressing aloofness, indifference, and a lack of caring.

ACTIVITY IV
Self-Reflection: Personal Traits of Caring

Write in detail about a caring encounter you have had with a patient. If you have not had a caring encounter with a patient, write about a caring experience in which you provided the care. The caring may range from comforting an emotionally upset acquaintance to caring for someone who was ill. Describe the following aspects of the experience.

1. What caring responses did you demonstrate?

2. How did you feel as a provider of care?

3. What were your greatest skills in providing care?

4. What skills do you need to develop to provide care?

5. Describe how the experience affected you.

6. Describe how the experience affected the recipient of your care.

7. What did you *not* do or say that you wished you had done or said? Why did you not do these things? What can you do differently next time?

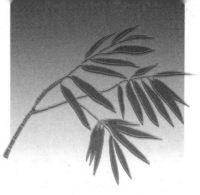

CHAPTER 5

Advocacy for Patients

Introduction

The role of the nurse as patient advocate is relatively new. Before the 1970s, the nurse's primary obligation was to carry out the physician's orders (Bernal, 1992). In 1940, the ANA's Tentative Code of Ethics noted that this obligation of "loyalty to the physician demands that the nurse conscientiously follow his instruction and that she build up the confidence of the patient in him" (Veins, 1989, p. 47). However, with the 1960s Civil Rights Movement and the consumer movement, the primary obligation of the nurse began to shift toward the patient. Thus the nurse's role as "client advocate" was described in the 1976 ANA Code revision: "The nurse must be alert to and take appropriate action regarding any instances of incompetent, unethical, or illegal practice(s) by any member of the health care team or the health care system itself, or any action on the part of others that is prejudicial to the client's best interest" (ANA Code, 1976, p. 9). This description of the nurse as advocate remained unchanged in the 1985 and 1997 draft of the Code of Ethics.

This chapter opens with a discussion of three aspects of patient advocacy:
- The moral significance of advocacy
- Patient advocacy roles
- Requirements of advocacy

The Moral Significance of Advocacy

The notion of patient advocacy is built on the assumption that patients have certain rights and health care providers have a duty to ensure that patients' rights are honored (Mallik, 1997). Patients are entitled to have their voices heard, but they are often unable to fend for themselves in the health care system because of the compromises of illness. Therefore, patients need an advocate.

The moral significance of patient advocacy lies in three linked concerns. First, when a patient's health is threatened, the patient faces a possible loss of quality of life, rendering situations in which health is threatened morally significant (Liaschenko, 1995). Therefore, whenever patients' health is compromised, they deserve a knowledgeable advocate to help restore health or prevent further decline. The moral significance of advocacy also comes from the vulnerability of patients to illness and death. All human beings potentially share this vulnerability. The nurse is connected with patients through this shared vulnerability, and it is morally unacceptable to ignore fellow sufferers. This is particularly true for health care providers, upon whom society has conferred a special status to help persons whose health is threatened (Liaschenko, 1995).

The inequality of power between the advocate and the patient is a third moral element of advocacy (Liaschenko, 1995). The advocate's power resides in her knowledge, role, health, and affiliation with the institution to which the patient has come for help. Capturing the double-edged nature of this power, Liaschenko writes: "The power to act for others in such conditions [illness] is an occasion not only for compassion and nobility of spirit, but also for evil in the form of abuse of power" (p. 3). A challenge for the advocate is to avoid the abuse of power by acting for the patient, not the institutionalized health care system.

It is relatively easy to advocate for a patient whose values are in concert with our values or the values of the health care system. Advocacy is much more challenging when the patient's values differ from our own. Classic examples of this include a nurse who believes abortion is wrong who is working with a patient undergoing an abortion or situations in which a nurse is caring for an AIDS patient who contracted the disease through IV drug use or sexual activity and the nurse believes the behaviors that led to the disease were wrong. In such situations the moral requirement is to recognize that a conflict in values may threaten compassionate care. With this awareness the nurse must either overcome the temptation to withhold care from the patient or, if someone else is available and willing to care for the patient, ask the other to assume responsibility for the patient's care. In situations when no one else is available to care for the patient, the nurse must provide competent, compassionate care.

Patient Advocacy Roles

Various authors have suggested that the nurse is the ideal patient advocate, and the ongoing and regular contact that nurses have with patients situates them best for advocacy (Winslow, 1984). Others think that the intimate care nurses provide patients and the knowledge nurses have of patients when they are most vulnerable position nurses to be advocates (Copp, 1986). Still others say that nurses should be patient advocates because their role situates them between the patient and physician, thus positioning them for advocacy (Mallik, 1997).

While there is little argument that nurses can be excellent patient advocates, ideally, *all* health care providers are patient advocates. Indeed, effective patient advocacy requires a team effort. In this regard, the responsibility of the nurse extends beyond advocacy for patients to collegial and reciprocal relationships with all members of the health care team. The shared decision making of team members promotes a form of advocacy in which patient needs are examined through the different lens of team members. For example, the nurse focuses on the response of the patient to illness; this view is complemented by the physician's perspective on diagnosis and treatment and the social worker's perspective on financial and discharge needs. A multidisciplinary team that works well together promotes shared advocacy and optimum patient outcomes (Sheer, 1996).

In most health care teams the case manager—usually a nurse or a social worker—coordinates health care services (Siefker, Garrett, Genderen, & Weis, 1998). Case managers may work in hospitals, rehabilitation facilities, home health agencies, or for employer groups, health maintenance organizations (HMOs), or major insurance companies. In case management, advocacy involves serving as liaison between the patient and the health care team or community, keeping the patient informed of the plan of care, and communicating the needs and wishes of the patient to the team (Cesta, Hahan, & Fink, 1998; Mullahy, 1998; Siefker et al., 1998). Case managers must balance the tension between quality and cost. In some situations, it is difficult to speak up for patients given the pressures to keep costs down. However, in the long run, both the organization and the patient are better served when the case manager accurately represents patient needs, regardless of cost, since faulty decisions that result in poor patient outcomes can and should be appealed, resulting in increased management costs (Siefker et al., 1998). Finally, the case manager must always remember that the patient, not the organization for which the case manager works, is the client (Cesta et al., 1998; Siefker et al., 1998).

Most nursing literature depicts the nurse advocate working directly with patients rather than at the broader level of the community. However, nurses may also be advocates at the community level when they work to influence public health policy or promote through political means the development of services for a population in need. Chapter 6 offers a discussion of population-focused advocacy.

Requirements of Advocacy

Advocacy can take many forms, depending upon the values and needs of the patient. Advocacy can be simple, requiring nothing more than getting an order for sufficient pain medication for a suffering patient, or it can be complex, as in helping a patient decide whether to undergo potentially life-saving but significantly risky chemotherapy. Recall Betsy's story in Chapter 2. Betsy demonstrated advocacy when she helped Mr. James realize his desire to stay at home as his congestive heart failure became worse. She supported his wish by making visits to his home and arranging for him to sleep in the living room so as not to disturb his wife. In a more dramatic way Eliese, in Chapter 1, advocated for a patient who refused a life-saving blood transfusion that conflicted with his beliefs as a Jehovah's Witness.

Envisioned broadly, advocacy may include planning and implementing nursing care, health promotion and disease prevention; caring for dying patients; and protecting patients who participate in research (Copp, 1986). Fundamentally, advocacy entails advising patients of their rights, providing information so patients can make informed decisions, and then supporting those decisions (Mallik, 1997). Advocacy also includes helping patients to clarify their values and make decisions that are compatible with the way they have lived their lives, thus helping patients maintain their personal integrity (Liaschenko, 1995). This may not be a simple or straightforward process since a patient's values often shift in response to illness. However, the advocate helps patients sort out shifting values by listening, providing information about the illness, and affirming the multiple aspects of the patient's experience.

The ANA Code of Ethics (1997) depicts advocacy broadly as a commitment "to the health, well-being, and safety of the patient across the life span and in all settings. . . . This includes not only those acts that prevent, promote, maintain, and restore health but also those that alleviate suffering and promote a peaceful, comfortable and dignified death" (p. 9). This broad view of advocacy requires finely developed skills that are acquired through experience and practice. The nurse must be familiar with the system in which he works in order to envision and actualize patient options (Snowball, 1996). Further, the nurse needs personal skills, including excellent listening skills, an ability to negotiate, tact, and confidence (Copp, 1986). These personal skills were depicted in Eliese's story in Chapter 1. When the physician ordered blood for the Jehovah's Witness patient who had refused a transfusion, she not only heard the doctor's order but also noted the physician's urgent wish to save the patient's life. Though she understood both, she steadfastly refused to give the blood against the patient's expressed wish. Her listening skills and tact were key to keeping communication open rather than creating a standoff with the physician in which no one, especially the patient, could win. Her confidence was critical to ensuring that the patient's values ruled and to preserving his integrity in the situation.

Eliese also demonstrated certain traits that enhance patient advocacy including assertiveness, persistence, and ethical awareness (Chafey, Rhea, Shannon, & Spencer, 1998). Other traits identified as bolstering advocacy are empathy and nurturance (Chafey et al., 1998). The nurse's empathetic response to the patient and recognition of the shared human experience of vulnerability often motivate the response of advocacy. Recall how Ben, in Chapter 1, recognized Mrs. Floyd's terror and need for reassurance when she began to bleed from her carotid artery. This recognition came from his empathetic awareness that he too would be frightened in such a situation.

It should be noted that patient advocacy is greatly facilitated by an environment that promotes patient self-determination. A management team that does not support the advocate can make advocacy impossible. However, whatever the nurse's level of skill or the degree of environmental support, there are ways in which nurses can initiate simple, humanizing activities on behalf of patients that support patient advocacy. For example, you can explain to patients what is going on, tell patients about changes in medications or treatments, pass patient concerns along to appropriate health care providers, and listen when patients share information about themselves.

Nurses and other members of the multidisciplinary team have key roles advocating for patients. The skills of advocacy are depicted in the story of Jana, whose knowledge of the system in which she worked and knowledge of the patient guided her advocacy for Margaret.

Jana's Story

Margaret was 43 years old when she first noticed pain in her abdomen. Not one to complain, she ignored the pain and the occasional blood in her stools as she continued to work in the textile mill where she had been employed for most of her life. Margaret knew how to press on when life was difficult. The oldest of four children of a single mom, she had dropped out of high school in the 10th grade and joined her mother in the mill to help support her family. She never married, but she had a daughter, who lived in a nearby town. When her mother became ill in her early fifties, Margaret took care of her for six months until she died.

When Margaret could no longer ignore her pain and had lost considerable weight, she went to the local doctor, who referred her to a medical center in a nearby city for further tests. A friend drove Margaret to her appointment with a surgeon. His examination and tests were alarming. Margaret's intestines were almost completely obstructed. Chiding her for not coming to him sooner, the surgeon told her he suspected cancer of the colon and admitted her to the hospital at once for abdominal surgery.

Jana had worked for seven years on the oncology floor to which Margaret was admitted. When Jana admitted Margaret, she found her to be like many of her patients—cooperative, scared about her surgery, largely ignorant about what was happening to her physically, and eager to please. Unlike some patients, however, Margaret spoke openly about her life and asked many questions about what was going to happen to her. Jana enjoyed teaching and explained what Margaret could expect before and after surgery. When Jana inquired whether any family member would be there during the surgery, Margaret answered, "No, my daughter cannot come."

Because of Margaret's severe weight loss, the doctor ordered total parenteral nutrition (TPN) in preparation for surgery. This allowed Margaret to receive nutritional support through her veins, bypassing her diseased intestines. Jana explained the purpose of the thick TPN solution. Having entirely lost her appetite and the ability to eat, Margaret expressed relief that she was now "getting food."

On the day of Margaret's surgery, Jana received Margaret from the operating room nurses. She was drowsy and in pain. Her vital signs were stable, but the report was not good: Margaret had cancer throughout her intestines that could not be surgically removed. At this late stage, neither chemotherapy nor radiation would help: nothing could be done to heal Margaret. The TPN was discontinued and comfort measures were to be initiated to sustain her through her dying. The surgeon would be around in a few hours to tell Margaret the grim outcome of the surgery. Jana felt sad. Margaret had faced many obstacles. Now, in her early forties, this spirited lady was dying.

Receiving regular doses of pain medication, Margaret slept fitfully until the surgeon arrived at about 6 PM. Jana went with him to see Margaret. The surgeon explained the situation to Margaret and concluded by assuring her they would do all they could to keep her comfortable during these last weeks of her life. Shaken and quiet, Margaret asked no questions. Jana stayed with her after the surgeon left. When she asked Margaret if she wanted to talk, Margaret shook her head, "No." Jana expressed to Margaret her sorrow at the surgical outcome and reassured Margaret that she would be there for her over the next weeks. Jana remembered thinking, She is my age. That could be me.

That evening, Jana checked Margaret's vital signs, dressing, and IV site; kept the IV fluids running; offered her pain medication, which Margaret accepted; and looked for any response to indicate how Margaret was taking the bad news. Margaret remained quiet and uncomplaining.

The next afternoon, a more alert Margaret noted that the TPN had been discontinued. She asked Jana why she was not "getting that food through my veins. I need that food to keep my strength up since I can't eat."

Jana asked Margaret, "What do you understand about the surgical findings?"

Without hesitation, Margaret replied, "I have bad cancer. There is nothing they can do to cure me. I am going to die. But I still want that food."

Jana explained the rationale for discontinuing TPN for patients who are dying: the nutrition prolongs the dying and consequently the patient's suffering and pain. Thus the burdens of TPN outweigh the benefits. She reassured Margaret that dying patients do not experience hunger and her IVs would provide hydration and minimum calories.

Margaret then explained why she wanted the TPN: "It's not that I'm afraid of dying, because I'm not. It's something else. My only daughter and I did not speak for over a year. We argued over her boyfriend. Two months ago I heard from friends that she was pregnant and I broke down and called her. For the last six weeks, we have been talking on the phone and she even came by the house once. We're finally becoming friends again. I want to live until she has the baby. She's due in five weeks. That's why I want the food."

Touched by her request, Jana talked with Margaret further about her desire to reinstate the TPN. She wanted to make sure Margaret understood fully the burdens and benefits of TPN in her situation.

"Do you understand that if you get the TPN your dying will be prolonged and your suffering may be greater?" Jana asked Margaret.

"Yes," Margaret replied, "I understand that. I only care about having more time with my daughter."

When Jana felt certain that Margaret understood the issues and still wanted the TPN, she suggested that Margaret ask the doctor to restart the nutritional support. Jana said, "I prefer that patients ask questions for themselves when they can. This gives them a greater sense of participation in health care decisions. I felt Margaret could handle this with my encouragement and guidance."

The next day a disappointed Margaret reported that the doctor had denied her request. He had insisted that TPN was not medically indicated. Margaret said there was little discussion. "He just didn't understand," she said.

Jana offered to speak to the surgeon on Margaret's behalf. When she did, she found the surgeon unrelenting. "No TPN for a dying patient," he said.

"It was like we were coming from two different planets," said Jana. "He believed that since Margaret could not get well and therefore would never be a productive member of society, it was a poor use of resources to give her TPN. He felt that resources like TPN should be used on persons who could recover. I simply could not see his point. The patient had requested TPN. Her wish for time to heal the broken relationship with her daughter was a valid reason for ordering the TPN. Her request deserved our support. Sure, it might prolong her dying and increase her suffering, but this was her wish. Besides, we could stop it at any point." Jana concluded, "The surgeon and I were both angry and neither of us was trying to understand the other. It was a real tug-of-war."

Frustrated and a little shaken by the confrontation with the surgeon, Jana next discussed the issue with fellow nurses and physicians, who supported her and her efforts for Margaret. Her nurse colleagues suggested she seek guidance from the unit nurse supervisor, who was sympathetic to patient needs.

The supervisor felt she could not be any more effective than Jana in dealing with this doctor. Recognizing that Margaret's surgeon was of the "old school" and believed that nurses were simply handmaidens to physicians, the supervisor suggested that perhaps the hospital ethics committee would be the best setting for resolving the standoff. Perhaps the surgeon would listen to his physician colleagues on the committee. So a plan was made for Jana to call the chair of the ethics committee that day and request a meeting as soon as possible.

Within hours the physician chair of the ethics committee returned Jana's call. Jana explained the situation as she understood it. Indeed, this sounded like an emergency to the chair of the committee, who said they could meet with 24 hours notice. Their general procedure was that the nurses caring for the patient, any family representatives, and the physicians involved would come to the meeting to present the case. The multidisciplinary ethics committee would then help resolve the issue. If the key players were available, they could meet the next day. The chair would contact the surgeon about the meeting. Jana asked the chair if she would talk with the surgeon and see if they might resolve the issue without having to take it to the ethics committee. "He might listen to you since you are a physician colleague. I would like to avoid a public confrontation in the ethics committee if possible," Jana explained.

Jana later said, "I was nervous. I don't like confrontations but I was willing to engage in a showdown with the surgeon if I had to. A nurse colleague was going to go with me for support. I simply could not let Margaret's request be brushed off. She needed me and I was in a position to help. Emotionally, it wasn't easy for me, but I received a lot of encouragement from my fellow nurses and from some of the doctors with whom I had talked. And of course, Margaret was foremost in my mind. This bolstered me. I have a daughter. I understood what she wanted."

Much to Jana's relief, the chair of the ethics committee called her later that evening to report that, after some discussion, the surgeon had volunteered to withdraw from the case. Margaret now needed a new physician.

A delighted Margaret heard Jana's report and asked Jana to find her a doctor. Jana reasoned that an oncologist would be familiar with the needs of dying patients and sympathetic to Margaret's situation. She contacted one in whom she had already confided about the situation, and he agreed to take the case. By the next morning, the TPN was reinstated.

Although Margaret's care was not technically complex, it required time-consuming, hands-on nursing. Margaret grew weaker each day and needed help with bathing, toileting, skin and mouth care. Each shift Jana and other nurses got her out of bed and propped her in the large chair in her room. Because of her intestinal obstruction, she had a gastrostomy tube inserted during surgery that drained the stomach contents into a bag affixed to her bed. This bag required emptying each shift and sometimes more often, since Margaret liked to sip juice that flowed directly from her stomach into the collection bag. Pain control was a balancing act as the nurses tried to keep her comfortable yet still alert. While it was clear that Margaret was in pain, she rarely complained.

Margaret's daughter became a frequent visitor. Several times a week she drove up from the nearby town where she lived with her boyfriend. She and her mother spent time talking and simply being together as they waited for the birth. Her daughter told her she had selected a name for the baby if it were a girl. She would be called Margaret.

Margaret grew increasingly weak and her pain escalated. Jana explained, "She declined rapidly, yet wanted badly to live until her grandbaby came. Many of the nurses and doctors became engaged in Margaret's story and asked about her each day. Even the chair of the ethics committee stopped by to ask about her every once in a while. Everyone was hoping she would make it until the delivery."

To ease her growing pain, Margaret was put on a morphine drip that allowed her to have continuous pain relief. At her request, the dosage was kept low enough so she could be alert for her daughter's visits.

One day her daughter brought Margaret a gift of three pairs of black lace bikini panties. She told her mother, "I know how you loved to wear black lace underwear." The nurses helped a pleased Margaret into the bikinis that just fit under the gastrostomy site.

Margaret's granddaughter was born without complications and was brought by the daughter and her boyfriend to meet Margaret when she was four days old. The nurses and several doctors crowded into the room to welcome the baby and congratulate an elated Margaret. Shortly after everyone except the family had left the room, Jana noticed through the cracked door that Margaret, her daughter, and the baby were all asleep in Margaret's bed. The reconciliation was complete.

Almost immediately after she met the baby, Margaret became weaker and her pain escalated. Margaret told Jana, "I'm in a lot of pain. My daughter and I are OK now. I'm leaving two beautiful girls in my place. I'm ready to die." Margaret concluded, "Could you help me die? Could you add something to my IV that would help me die quickly?"

Jana recalled, "Her request was no less genuine than her earlier plea for TPN. I understood her feelings. She was dying slowly and had endured great pain. She had reconciled with her daughter and held the baby. With typical courage and clarity, she knew what she wanted and she asked for it. But I could not help her die that way. It would have been illegal and, besides, the nursing profession does not support the nurse's participation in euthanasia. I could, however, make her comfortable."

Explaining her position to Margaret, Jana offered other options. They could discontinue the TPN, withdrawing this form of sustenance. The morphine could be increased to better control her pain, though not with the intention of killing her. Jana reminded Margaret that as the morphine was increased, her respirations would slow down and her ability to communicate with others would diminish. Margaret asked that the TPN be stopped and said that if she could hold out that long, she wanted to wait for maximum pain control until after her daughter and baby visited one more time.

Jana called the oncologist, and by evening the TPN was discontinued and the order for morphine had been changed to allow the nurses to increase the dose as Margaret's pain control needs dictated. The next day, after a visit with her daughter and baby Margaret, Margaret told Jana, "I'm ready now for more morphine."

Because of Margaret's pain, it was increasingly difficult for the nurses and Margaret to negotiate using the bedpan. Jana suggested to Margaret that they insert a Foley catheter so that she would not have to struggle when she needed to void. Margaret resisted, "I don't mind using the bedpan," she said. "I don't want a catheter. I want to die in my black bikini panties." Later Jana recalled, "The decision not to use a Foley during the last days of her life was hard for some of the other nurses to understand. It created more work for all of us and seemed hard on Margaret. But this was what Margaret wanted. I had to talk to the other nurses to get them to go along with the plan, but since I was the primary nurse, they respected what I had set out to do for Margaret. Thankfully, despite heavy doses of morphine, Margaret never became incontinent. If she had become incontinent, I think we probably would have had to put in a Foley. I was so glad we didn't have to do that."

Margaret died in her black bikini panties. Her granddaughter was one week old. Jana remembered Margaret fondly: "Margaret was one of a kind. She had a lot of courage and spirit. She set about to get what she deserved and wanted. It never occurred to her that I wouldn't help her. And it never occurred to me not to help her. There was something about Margaret that grabbed me and I just couldn't turn away. I had to help her get what she deserved."

Enacting Artful Nursing

Jana's familiarity with the system in which she worked including the personalities of her physician and nurse colleagues, along with her knowledge of the care of oncology patients, a supportive work environment, and an empathetic connection to her patient provided a foundation for her advocacy on behalf of Margaret. Jana's story illustrates four aspects of advocacy:
- A focus on the patient
- Awareness of patient rights

- Honoring patient values
- Activities of advocacy

A FOCUS ON THE PATIENT

It is surprising how easy it is to overlook patient needs in a busy nursing practice. Recognizing opportunities for advocacy requires engaged, patient-centered care (Chafey et al., 1998; Snowball, 1996). Nothing, including equipment, the doctor's orders, treatment goals, or even the nursing care plan, must distort the nurse's vision of the patient as the focus of care. Jana's attention to Margaret was key to recognizing and respecting Margaret's need for an advocate. If she had not recognized the validity of Margaret's request, she would not have helped Margaret continue TPN. Jana remained Margaret's advocate to the end, encouraging Margaret to decide when to discontinue the TPN, when to increase the morphine, and even whether to insert a Foley catheter.

When the nurse's attention is on the patient, she begins to understand the patient. As Jana listened to Margaret's story, she recognized that Margaret valued relationships—evidenced in her caring for her dying mother and her current wish to heal the broken relationship with her daughter. She also noted that Margaret had spunk; she did not let her limited education and lack of sophistication thwart her perseverance in asking for what she needed and wanted. Jana's understanding strengthened Jana's identification with Margaret as a fellow human being. It never occurred to Jana not to advocate for Margaret. "That could have been me," she mused. Recognizing her patient's vulnerability, Jana concluded, "She needed help and I could help her." Her advocacy thus flowed from her personal involvement: "I just couldn't turn away," she recalled. Jana's advocacy was based on skills in engaging with and getting to know her patient and was stimulated by an empathetic response to Margaret's situation.

AWARENESS OF PATIENT RIGHTS

Recognizing and honoring patient rights are essential to patient advocacy. Her knowledge of Margaret's right to request TPN led Jana to inform Margaret of that right and then to help her actualize the right. The surgeon's refusal to reinstate the TPN, based upon a teleological framework (see Chapter 3) that supported his belief that a greater good would be achieved by using medical resources for patients with the potential for health, was an ethically sound argument. Clearly the physician felt Margaret's request exceeded the limits of patient rights.

And indeed, there are limits to patient rights. Jana recognized this when Margaret asked for her help to die. Jana's refusal was based upon both legal constraints and professional nursing values that prohibit active euthanasia. Yet regardless of whether she agreed with Margaret's requests, her support for her patient did not waver. Although she refused to help Margaret die, she offered suggestions for palliative care such as stopping the TPN and increasing pain control.

HONORING PATIENT VALUES

Effective advocacy requires knowledge of the patient's values. Respect for patient values ensures the patient's right to be self-determined and helps the patient find personal meaning in the illness experience. For example, extending Margaret's dying so that she could reconcile with her daughter gave significant meaning to the experience. Her suffering was worthwhile because it allowed a renewed relationship with her daughter. Once the reconciliation was complete and the grandchild was safely born, the meaning of her suffering was fulfilled. She was ready to die. She could say with satisfaction, "I am leaving two beautiful girls in my place."

Honoring patient values sustains the integrity of the patient (Liaschenko, 1995). Because Margaret's wishes were honored, she died as she had lived, facing with courage what she had to face, reconciled with her daughter and in her black lace bikinis. While honoring her values gave Margaret a sense of self-determination, more significantly it preserved her identity and uniqueness.

Patient values are most frequently ascertained by simply listening. Jana did not need extended contact with Margaret to discern her values. As Margaret described quitting high school to help support her family, caring for her dying mother, and experiencing pain because of the broken relationship with her daughter, Jana noted the centrality of family relationships to her patient. This awareness was reinforced by Margaret's willingness to prolong her suffering and dying with TPN in order to have time to reconcile with her daughter and meet her grandchild.

In some cases advocacy involves helping a patient reevaluate personal values (Gadow, 1980). Illness is a powerful disruption of the life of a patient. Illness occasions reflection during which values are reconsidered and in some cases realigned. For example, though Margaret acknowledged her sadness over the broken relationship with her daughter, so long as her health was good she did not give priority to reconciliation. However, when she realized she was dying, the value of mending the relationship took priority over everything, including her own suffering. Jana helped Margaret consider her values by providing information about her physical condition and discussing with her the benefits and burdens of TPN so she could make informed choices.

The surgeon's refusal to honor Margaret's request for TPN and Jana's refusal to help Margaret die illustrate the difficulty in advocating for patients whose values are in conflict with the personal or professional values of the advocate. In situations such as these, a patient-centered approach in which patient needs are acknowledged, along with the professional or personal constraints of the nurse, guide the advocate. In these situations, advocacy may entail finding another professional to care for the patient, as Jana did for Margaret.

ACTIVITIES OF ADVOCACY

Advocacy for Margaret included direct interventions as well as negotiation within the organization. Jana advised Margaret of her rights and gave her the information she needed to make informed decisions. She taught Margaret about the burdens and benefits of TPN and made sure Margaret understood. She provided adequate pain control and kept her patient comfortable. Jana encouraged Margaret to act on her own behalf when she could, suggesting she ask the surgeon to reinstate the TPN. When Margaret met obstacles she could not handle on her own—when the surgeon refused to restart the TPN or she wanted the TPN discontinued and to die in her bikinis—Jana stepped in as her spokesperson.

Jana's ability to advocate for Margaret at the system level required knowledge of the organization in which she worked. Having functioned in the setting for seven years, Jana understood the roles of the various professionals and who might best help her patient achieve her goals. She knew possible options for her patient, the chain of command to follow to get help, the challenges of working with certain colleagues, and the people to turn to for her own support and support for Margaret. Jana knew that the climate in which she worked was basically supportive of patient rights; this greatly facilitated her efforts to find persons in the environment who could help her patient.

It is not unusual for nurses to experience fear, fatigue, frustration, and burnout when acting as advocates. These feelings are related to the many obstacles to nurse advocacy, including a hierarchical structure in which nurses have less power than physicians (Chafey et al., 1998). Jana's talk with the surgeon was characterized by anger, little effort to understand his position, and dislike of confrontations. Yet despite her fears of confrontation and the impediments imposed by the surgeon, Jana was persistent. Persistence has been identified by nurses as "a significant contributor to successful advocacy" (Chafey et al., 1998, p. 49). When her efforts with the surgeon failed, Jana took two important steps: (1) she turned to her nurse and physician colleagues for support and (2) she sought guidance about how to proceed from her immediate supervisor and continued to work within the system until the TPN was reinstated.

Jana's recognition of her own strengths and limitations was central to her success. She knew her professional capabilities, and despite her anxiety about confrontation, she did not relinquish her advocacy role in the face of physician resistance. Recognizing that she could not win in a power struggle with the surgeon, she asked the chair of the ethics committee to speak to him on Margaret's behalf. This spared her further conflict with the surgeon and helped get the needed TPN for her patient in a timely fashion.

Jana's advocacy was based on knowledge of her patient's values, awareness of her patient's vulnerability and need for an advocate, and skills in enacting advocacy. There are, however, many challenges to advocacy by nurses, some of which are system driven and can thwart even the most skillful efforts at advocacy.

Challenges to Patient Advocacy

One of the major obstacles to patient advocacy, either as a case manager or as a nurse providing direct care, is that you will have multiple and at times conflicting obligations—to patient, physician, and institution. These conflicting loyalties have been complicated in recent years by managed care, which is not client centered but is driven by cost curtailments (Chafey et al., 1998). While conflicts are most evident in the role of case managers, who are often hired by insurance companies or organizations to help keep costs down, nurses providing direct patient care also report that organizational constraints, including economic and political concerns, sometimes prohibit effective advocacy. A nurse in a 1996 study suggested that "You have to weigh up not only what is in the patient's best interests, but what you can manage within the system" (Snowball,

p. 73). Nurses in Snowball's study complained that they were easily over-whelmed by the culture of "management" and had to take care not to "lose the vision of what we ought to be pursuing professionally" (p. 73).

Clearly nurses must work within very real system constraints. This is especially true in settings where every resource used requires a doctor's order if the organization is to be reimbursed. Learning to work within these constraints without losing sight of the patient calls for creative problem solving and sometimes hard choices by the nurse. You will not always be able to do everything you want to do for your patient. It is important, however, to recognize the constraints and speak on behalf of your patient whenever possible, in order to make others aware of the tension between patient and system needs.

Another impediment to patient advocacy is difficulties with other team members. As in the conflict Jana had with Margaret's surgeon, it is easy for struggles to emerge in which two perspectives are in conflict. You will quickly learn from peers and through experience how to work with a variety of personalities on multidisciplinary teams. In most cases, teams work well together. In cases of conflict, it may be useful to get support from sympathetic colleagues, as Jana did. Remember, however, that Jana's unwillingness to try to see the surgeon's perspective, while understandable, did not help her move toward a dialogue that might have led to mutual understanding and prompt resolution of the problem.

Awareness of patient rights entails constant acknowledgment of our commonalties with patients, including feelings of fear, vulnerability, dependence, and pain. Recognition that the patient is a human being who has rights flows from this. It is easy, however, to forget this when the demands of practice bring on fatigue and burnout. Awareness of commonalties with patients may also be hindered by differences between you and your patients in culture, socioeconomic status, knowledge, or power. However, when we do not remember our human connection with patients, we forget both our patients and ourselves and fall back on automatic, unfeeling responses.

One way to remember the human connection with patients is to find something you have in common with your patient such as being a student, or a mother, or a lover, or sick, or happy, or courageous, or afraid. There is *always* some human experience or feeling we have in common with patients. Recognition of ourselves in our patients through acknowledging shared feelings or experiences closes the gap between provider and patient that is so easily created in a busy health care situation.

With patients like Margaret who openly talk about themselves, discovering patient values is easy. There are, however, many patients who are reluctant to talk about themselves. In these cases, you may need to ask directly and often, What is important to you in this experience? or What do you want in this experience? When patients are unable to talk because of their illness, family members and friends can help the nurse know what the patient might want in a particular situation. In those cases when patients simply do not wish to talk to the nurse, these wishes should be respected.

There will be circumstances in which you will not share the patient's goals or values. In such cases, patient values and goals overrule those of the nurse, except when patient values are incompatible with medical possibilities, available resources, or professional values. For example, when a patient is dying yet requests full life-support in an intensive care unit, that patient would take a bed that may be needed by someone with potential for full recovery. Some believe that the patient's values would not be compatible with medical possibilities or a just distribution of the scarce resource of intensive care unit beds. When the patient's wishes conflict with our values but are otherwise ethical and feasible, the challenge is to rise above our own resistance and honor patient values.

In addition to these challenges to the activities of advocacy, fear may obstruct advocacy efforts. It can be frightening to speak up for a patient. To do so is to single one's self out from others and to risk looking naive or ill informed. Indeed, it may be difficult for you to speak up in your nursing classes or clinical conferences. Fear presents the greatest problem when it goes unrecognized and silences nurses without their awareness. Hence, to overcome reluctance to speak up for yourself or your patients, it is useful to acknowledge your fear, without self-blame, and to face your anxiety. It is often effective to ask for help from a supportive colleague. You may also find it beneficial to practice speaking up in situations that are relatively safe, such as a familiar clinical or classroom setting when you can trust that you will be heard without ridicule. Experience is an excellent teacher. As you begin to learn when and how to speak up for patients, your skills will grow and your fears subside.

Effective advocacy can be thwarted by an approach that is belligerent or contentious. When your efforts on behalf of patients are met with opposition, as was the case with Margaret's surgeon, it is natural to feel anger on behalf of the patient. However, as in Jana's example, anger at another team member most often moves the nurse away from the goal. Using the energy of anger to fuel problem solving rather than attacking a team member is much more likely to accomplish your aims.

Mutual understanding is key to avoiding antagonism in advocacy efforts. Recall in Chapter 3 how David and the team came to the meeting with Lois with different perspectives about when Chip should be taken off the ventilator. As they talked and listened, they reached mutual understanding and resolved the dilemma without acrimony. In David's example, *mutual* understanding was key. Had Jana and the surgeon tried to understand each other's position, they might have resolved the disagreement without going to the ethics committee.

Finally, there will be times when you will overlook the patient's need. You cannot always be alert to every patient need, nor can you always be in synch with your patients. What you can do is learn to recognize and accept your human limitations in this regard and notice when your vision is not on the patient. Recognizing the need for advocacy is the first step; learning how to be an effective advocate comes with experience and practice.

Summary

Jana's advocacy was built upon her knowledge of pathophysiology, the requirements of palliative care, self-knowledge about her aversion to confrontations and her need for personal support, information about the system in which she worked, and knowledge of her patient, including the patient's values and responses to her illness. A patient who revealed what she valued and a work setting that was sympathetic to patient-centered decision making strengthened Jana's efforts at advocacy. The development of advocacy skills starts with personal knowledge of yourself, knowledge of your patient, and an understanding of the system in which you work. Advocacy skills can then be cultivated by watching others acting as patient advocates and by practice.

References

ANA code of ethics. (1976). Kansas City, MO: American Nurses' Association.

Bernal, E.W. (1992). The nurse as patient advocate. *Hastings Center Report, 22*(4), 18–23.

Cesta, T.G., Hahan, H.A., & Fink, L.F. (1998). *The case manager's survival guide.* St. Louis: Mosby.

Chafey, K., Rhea, M., Shannon, A.M., & Spencer, S. (1998). Characterizations of advocacy by practicing nurses. *Journal of Professional Nursing, 14,* 43–52.

Copp, L.A. (1986). The nurse as advocate for vulnerable persons. *Journal of Advanced Nursing, 11,* 225–263.

Gadow, S. (1980). Existential advocacy: Philosophical foundation of nursing. In S.F. Spicker & S. Gadow (Eds.), *Nursing: Images and ideals.* New York: Springer Publishing Company.

Liaschenko, J. (1995). Ethics in the work of acting for patients. *Advances in Nursing Science, 18*(2), 1–12.

Mallik, M. (1997). Advocacy in nursing—a review of the literature. *Journal of Advanced Nursing, 23,* 130–138.

Mullahy, C.M. (1998). *The case manager's handbook.* Gaithersburg, MD: Aspen Publishers, Inc.

Sheer, B. (1996). Reaching collaboration through empowerment: A developmental process. *Journal of Obstetric, Gynecologic, and Neonatal Nursing, 25,* 513–517.

Siefker, J.M., Garrett, M.B., Genderen, A.V., & Weis, M.J. (1998). *Fundamentals of case management.* St. Louis: Mosby.

Snowball, J. (1996). Asking nurses about advocating for patients: 'Reactive' and 'proactive' accounts. *Journal of Advanced Nursing, 24,* 67–73.

Veins, D.C. (1989). A history of nursing's code of ethics. *Nursing Outlook, 37,* 45–49.

Willard, C. (1996). The nurse's role as patient advocate: Obligation or imposition? *Journal of Advanced Nursing, 24,* 60–68.

Winslow, G.R. (1984). From loyalty to advocacy: A new metaphor for nursing. *Hastings Center Report,* June, 32–40.

APPLICATION

ACTIVITY I
Group Discussion: Analysis of the Story

Imagine you are the nurse caring for Margaret.

1. What would you have said when Margaret asked why she was not "getting that food through my veins" and then declared, "I need that food to keep my strength up since I can't eat"? What are the reasons for your response?

2. Jana sought help and support from colleagues, her supervisor, and ultimately the ethics committee at the hospital. Can you think of other ways she might have been able to resolve the conflict she was having with the physician?

3. What would you have said when Margaret asked you, "Could you help me die?" What reasons would you give for your answer. Discuss whether you think it is ever appropriate for a nurse to help a terminal patient who is suffering die. State your reasons for your answer.

4. What would you have done when Margaret said she did not want the Foley catheter? How would you explain your choice not to insert a catheter to your colleagues who had to work harder because Margaret did not have a Foley catheter? How would you explain your choice to insert a Foley catheter to Margaret?

ACTIVITY II
Case Analysis with Group Discussion:
Advocating for Patients

You are caring for an 86-year-old woman, Mrs. Morris. Since her husband died 20 years ago, Mrs. Morris has lived alone. She has managed well in her small house. She has no children. A neighbor has done her weekly shopping, and she has used a local transportation service for trips to the physician.

Mrs. Morris was admitted to the hospital with a severe infection secondary to a blister on her foot that did not heal. It has been determined that she has diabetes, and she now has gangrene in her foot. She needs an amputation below the knee. She is alert and oriented. Reluctantly she has agreed to the surgery, having signed a consent form that was presented by her physician.

You are a relatively new nurse, having worked for eight months. You are caring for Mrs. Morris. When you do her preoperative teaching, you find she is upset. She has decided she does not want the surgery. You explain to her that it is unlikely she will recover without surgery since the gangrene will spread. Her response is immediate. She explains that she knows that. She has lived a wonderful, long life and is ready to die. Her preference is to die rather than have surgery, lose her foot, and have to go to a nursing home to live. She concludes by stating that if it can be arranged, she would like to go home and die. If that cannot be arranged, she says that she will die here in the hospital. She states that under no circumstances will she have her foot amputated.

There is no reason to question her mental competence. She is alert, oriented, and understands the consequences of her choice. She is clear about what she wants. You call the surgeon and report what you have found. Her response is that the patient has already signed the consent and is just having normal presurgical fears. She instructs you to follow through with the preoperative preparations. The surgery is scheduled for the next morning.

GROUP DISCUSSION QUESTIONS

1. Discuss how you would feel in this situation: Angry? Afraid? Powerful? Helpless? Confused? Conflicted?

2. Time is pressing. Whatever you do must be done during this shift. Describe what you think might be your options. How would you go about acting on these options? Who do you think could help you?

3. Discuss obstacles to patient advocacy in the various clinical settings in which you have had experience. Are some settings more supportive of nurse advo-

cacy efforts than others? If so, what do you think contributes to the differences in settings?

4. Discuss the differences among nurses in regard to advocacy efforts. What characteristics of effective advocates have you seen in your clinical experiences?

ACTIVITY III
Group Activity: Seeking Understanding

The purpose of this activity is to help students practice engaging in dialogue around an advocacy issue.

Divide into two groups. Groups 1 and 2 will engage in dialogue about whether Margaret should be given TPN. Group 1 will represent the position of the surgeon in Jana's story. Recall that he did not want to give Margaret TPN because he felt the resource of TPN should be used for patients who could benefit from it. This is a sound ethical argument, based on a teleological framework. (See Chapter 3 for clarification of teleology.)

Group 2 will represent Jana's position. Recall that Jana believed Margaret's request for TPN was legitimate based upon her wish to heal the broken relationship with her daughter. Jana's position is a sound ethical position that is supported by the ethic of care. (See Chapter 3 for clarification of ethic of care.)

Allow 15 minutes for the two groups to talk to each other with the intention of trying to reach a compromise in regard to Margaret's care.

GROUP DISCUSSION QUESTIONS

1. Was it difficult to reach a compromise?

2. Do you think Margaret's best interest was primary in the compromise?

3. How did you feel: Understood? Angry? Frustrated? Diminished? Powerful?

4. Describe the extent to which you were able to listen to the comments of the opposing group. Did you already have your mind made up about what was right in this situation?

5. Were you inclined to try to understand the other position? Were you listening, or were you thinking about how you might convince the other group that you were right?

6. Identify and describe your strengths and weakness in terms of the skills of advocacy.

ACTIVITY IV
Self-Reflection: Advocacy Skills

Assertiveness is behavior that helps you act in your own or the patient's best interest. Ideally assertive behavior does not create undue anxiety and allows you to express your ideas and feelings honestly without attacking the other person. Many individuals need to develop their assertive skills.

Complete the following sentences:

1. If I had been Jana, I would have

2. The hardest part of the experience for me would have been

3. My strengths in the area of patient advocacy are

4. My limitations in the area of patient advocacy are

5. The steps I might take to be more assertive are

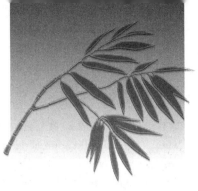

CHAPTER 6

Advocacy for Populations

··

Introduction

In 1893, a nurse named Lillian Wald was teaching in a neighborhood school when a ragged child approached her to tell of her sick mother. Troubled by the girl's account, Wald followed her through the crowded, dirty streets where children were playing to a tenement house. Entering the two-room apartment occupied by the seven members of the little girl's family and two boarders, Wald found a woman who had given birth lying on a bed soiled by a hemorrhage. She cleaned the woman and the newborn, whereupon the woman kissed her hands in gratitude. Wald wrote,

> That morning's experience was a baptism of fire. . . . When early morning found me still awake, my naïve conviction remained that, if people knew things—and 'things' meant everything implied in the condition of this family—such horrors would cease to exist, and I rejoiced that I had had a training in the care of the sick that itself would give me an organized relationship to the neighborhood in which this awakening had come (1971, pp. 8, 9).

Responding to this experience, Wald and another nurse, Mary Brewster, established the Henry Street Settlement House, and organized public health nursing was born in the United States. The first public health nurses provided a range of services to individuals, families, and communities. They also exposed to public scrutiny the social and economic problems associated with illness and disease (Thomas, 1999). Caring for the poor in homes, workplaces, schools, on street corners—wherever the disenfranchised lived and needed nursing services, these public health nurses offered direct care to individuals and families while promoting collective political action to improve the health of the community (Thomas, 1999).

Nurses continue this tradition today, practicing as clinicians, advocates, consultants, educators, collaborators, case managers, and researchers in community-based settings including patient homes, health departments, neighborhood schools, industrial or business environments, and correctional facilities. In these varied settings, community health nurses provide comprehensive health care and serve as advocates for individuals, families, groups, and communities (Hitchcock, Schubert, & Thomas, 1999).

This chapter will focus on the role of advocacy in community health nursing. Three aspects of community advocacy will be highlighted.

- Populations as the focus
- Cultural awareness
- Community partnerships

Populations as the Focus

Nursing education focuses primarily on caring for individual patients or families, with a limited focus on caring at the group or community level (Bent, 1999; Williams, 1997). This is also the case with many community health nursing courses, which focus on individuals or families within the community rather than on the community as a whole (Williams, 1997). Many of these courses do not always examine the role of nurse advocacy in the community, despite the widely accepted assumption that advocacy is central to effective community-focused nursing. Nevertheless, community- or population-focused advocacy is a focal point of nursing concern (Bent, 1999; Hitchcock et al., 1999; Spradley & Allender, 1997).

In community health nursing, patients or clients include populations. In Wald's day, the focus of the nurse in the community was on alleviating sanitation concerns or crowded living conditions. Today, the nurse might focus on teenage pregnancy or drug use. Regardless of the concern, the focus of advocacy efforts is populations, which may be conceptualized in a variety of ways. For example, populations may be groups of persons who are at risk and share similar characteristics, such as diabetics, migrant workers, or teenage mothers (Kang, 1995). Populations may also be defined by location or mutual interdependence, like an inner-city neighborhood (Bent, 1999). Regardless of the composition of the target population, community-based advocacy is comprehensive and ongoing (as opposed to episodic); it spans all age groups, health problems, and potential health problems; and it has a strong interdisciplinary component. Therefore, the role of the nurse in the community offers opportunities to "reflect the true breadth, depth, and potential of nursing practice" (Bent, 1999, p. 30).

Advocacy for communities differs from the advocacy for individuals described in Jana's story (Chapter 5). This difference in part reflects the focus on populations, as described above. Another difference lies in the fact that advocacy on behalf of populations occurs in communities, not in the traditional health delivery settings that are familiar to most nurses (Gadow & Schroeder, 1996). Further, within these communities, there are entrenched political and social agendas, ruling classes and disenfranchised persons, different cultural values among groups of persons, and differences in power and knowledge between the nurse and the population group needing advocacy, all of which create challenges for the nurse advocate (Bent, 1999). In short, advocacy for populations is complex: the advocate must attend to the multiple voices in the population and validate the experience of members of the population with an aim of "uncovering and changing unhealthy structures and situations . . . that threaten the community now and in its future" (Bent, 1999, p. 32).

The focus of advocacy efforts with populations is broad, encompassing three levels of care. Primary prevention, designed to prevent disease or disability, involves activities like teaching mothers about caring for children or helping low-income high school graduates learn interviewing skills for jobs. Secondary prevention includes activities related to early detection and treatment of disease and may include screening for hearing or vision problems, for example, in order to help individuals receive early diagnosis and treatment. Tertiary prevention is directed toward preventing disability and involves working with populations with chronic conditions such as children with disabilities or persons with AIDS (Kang, 1995). Community-focused advocacy may also entail engagement in politically directed undertakings to affect public health policy.

Cultural Awareness

Regardless of the population served, effective advocacy for populations begins with cultural awareness. This means that the nurse is sensitive to issues of diversity and uses culturally appropriate approaches in working with populations (Drew, 1996; Kavanagh, Absalom, Beil, & Schliessmann, 1999). There is always a risk that the nurse advocate whose efforts are designed to help others will actually widen the gulf between herself and the target population. This occurs when advocacy efforts do not reflect the values of the population. When a nurse approaches a population with an attitude of arrogance or judgment, or with an assumption that the nurse knows better than the members of the population the best approach or even the most pressing need, the nurse creates separation between herself and the population (Kavanagh et al., 1999). Such an approach is based upon an outdated notion that the health beliefs and practices of the professional should prevail over the cultural values of the target population: this approach not only fails to meet the needs of the population but also dismisses their values (Kavanagh et al., 1999). For example, reflecting on her experience with the Lakota population (a Native American population), a nurse observed, "I came thinking I could help the Lakota by doing 'good' here. I see now how arrogant that was on my part" (Kavanagh et al., 1999, p. 20).

Successful community advocacy begins with understanding, honoring, and preserving cultural health-related beliefs and practices. This requires understanding and affirmation of values and orientations that may differ from one's own. For example, in the Lakota culture, relationships and being with people are highly valued. The harried nurse who attends to all the details of health promotion but fails to take time to visit and talk with individual persons violates the values of the population and jeopardizes health promotion efforts.

Few nurses currently have the cultural competence required to work effectively with different cultural groups (Kavanagh et al., 1999). In part, that is because of the growing diversity of populations in this country. More fundamentally, however, it is because cultural competence, like nursing skills, depends upon experience within a culture and cannot be gained by simply reading about a culture. To work effectively with populations, the nurse must spend time with individuals within the population. The ability to provide culturally sensitive care is "directly related to the investment of time and commitment to establishing and pursuing meaningful dialogue" with the individuals comprising a given population (Kavanagh et al., 1999, p. 13).

One effective model for gaining cultural competence and strengthening advocacy is the partnership model, which sets the stage for the nurse and members of the population to learn from each other.

Community Partnerships

Partnerships with communities offer a useful approach to providing culturally sensitive care and strengthening advocacy possibilities (Gadow & Schroeder, 1996; Hitchcock et al., 1999). Partnerships are built upon the assumption of equality between members of the population and the nurse and recognize that "true expertise regarding health resides in the community itself" (Gadow & Schroeder, 1996, p. 132) and not entirely with the professional. As the nurse spends time within the community, he uncovers the community's health-related values and needs. For example, in many communities, families headed by single mothers are increasingly the norm. Without recognition of this, the nurse might overlook the health care needs of single mothers and their babies. By placing this vulnerable group out of the reach of health care efforts, advocacy efforts would fail (Gadow & Schroeder, 1996).

Partnerships confront the tendency to focus on the expertise and influence of the professional at the expense of the authority and self-determination of the population (Willis, Biggins, & Donovan, 1999). In true partnerships, all voices carry equal legitimacy. This is illustrated in Milio's classic book, *9226 Kercheval* (1970), in which she described her efforts to work in partnership with a disenfranchised community in the inner city of Detroit. Milio, a young Caucasian female, set out to establish a day-care center in concert with an inner-city African-American community in the 1970s.

At the time, tension between the races frequently ruptured into riots, and militants from both races raged again each other. Reflecting her understanding of the reciprocal nature of partnerships, Milio portrayed the influence of the population on her own understanding: "They were going to teach me, unwittingly, to see them not just as idealized symbols of the tragedy for which my white world was to blame, but as individuals unique in their subculture as I was in mine; and as individuals, too, sharing with me the physical, sensual, existential qualities common to all human beings" (p. 32). Persisting in her efforts to establish and maintain a working partnership with this community, Milio concluded, "Finally, I knew that if the project did not really involve the people in the neighborhood, if it did not become what they wanted, then it would be a failure. . . . [S]o *they* had to struggle to shape it and I with them for while. *Then* it would be theirs" (pp. 29, 31).

A significant feature of partnerships with communities is that, as dialogue develops, private issues such as birth control, abortion, domestic or child abuse, alcoholism, and drug use are brought into the public domain for discussion. For example, a nurse working in an inner city who sees a relationship between poverty and depression in young mothers might take an active role in lobbying for better mental health care for the underserved. In this process, the conversations about the matter of poverty and depression in young mothers shifts from the private to the public domain and the voice of disenfranchised populations may be heard for the first time (Gadow & Schroeder, 1996). Thus, the disempowered are empowered and individuals outside the community who are willing to hear are enlightened.

Nancy's story demonstrates her partnership and advocacy efforts with a rural, southern African-American community. Her story covers 25 years, beginning in the mid-1960s when segregation of the races and discrimination against African Americans were still widely practiced in the rural South. Nancy's exemplary advocacy on behalf of African-American women was stimulated by her own encounters as an African-American with a health system that was unresponsive and indifferent to her needs. Her advocacy efforts, sustained by her commitment to serve poor women, resulted in the creation of public clinics to meet the health care needs of women and children in her state.

Nancy's Story

In the mid-1960s Nancy was working as a licensed practical nurse (LPN) in a university-affiliated hospital. She had married at the age of 15, and after completing high school and starting her family, she became an LPN. She had known firsthand the burden of being poor and the frustrations of discrimination, and she was determined to overcome both. But her desire for a better life was not entirely self-serving. Nancy also wanted to help other poor women. She recalled how as a young mother waiting for health care in the free clinic, "I felt in my heart that it needed to be different. I wanted to make it different for other young women. I was from a very poor background, and I had been herded into a waiting room, where I sat all morning, often with my children, passing the time until I was seen by a resident or a student. Because of this experience, I wanted to change the situation for as many women as I could. I believed then, and I believe now, that regardless of what color you are or how much money you have, health care should be equal. I wanted to make that happen somewhere. I knew early what my challenge in life would be, and I just stepped up to the bat."

With Nancy's husband supporting her efforts, Nancy arranged to work part time and return to school. She explained, "I knew I needed to be competent and credible if I was going to help others. So the first thing I did was get more education." She completed her undergraduate work in nursing and went directly into a master's program, where she specialized in women's health. "I had a wonderful educational experience. I worked in local health departments (HD) with a nurse midwife, who was also one of my instructors. She taught me how to provide excellent and thorough care to women." Eventually Nancy became a clini-

cal nurse specialist (CNS), which qualified her, with physician backup, to see patients. "All I needed was a job and medical backup," she explained.

While in graduate school, Nancy had written a proposal for establishing
clinics served by master's prepared nurses and designed to help low-income
women. She recalled, "In the mid-70s, there were lots of grants available to
help the underserved. Somehow that little proposal got into the hands of someone at the university-based hospital where I had continued to work while I was
in school and soon I had an interview." A team of physicians in the department
of pediatrics in the medical school had just received a large grant to establish
pediatric clinics in a five-county region. The intent of the clinics was to combat
the high infant mortality rate in the state. Nancy, the team believed, would be
the perfect individual to set up these clinics. The fact that Nancy's specialty was
women's health, not pediatrics, was no problem for the physicians. They
promised that if she took the job, later on they would help her establish similar
clinics to serve the mothers of the pediatric patients. "We will work with you if
you will help us start these clinics," the team promised. As an employee of the
university hospital, Nancy was to go into local health departments, set up the
clinics, and teach the staff the skills needed to care for the patients.

About a year after beginning her new job, Nancy had an experience that
cemented her resolve to help underserved women. As she prepared to leave for
work one morning, she received a call from a nurse at one of the health departments where she was working asking Nancy if she could stop by a patient's
home on her way into work to check on her newborn child. Nancy knew the patient from the health department. She was a woman in her late 20s who now
had six children. She knew this pregnancy had been difficult. The patient's he-
moglobin (red blood count) had been dangerously low, and she was thin and
sick the entire pregnancy. Nancy hoped this pregnancy would be her last. Previously, when the husband had come with his family to the pediatric clinic,
Nancy had talked with him about birth control. Her hope had been that when
this child was born, he would consent to his wife having a bilateral tubal liga-
tion (BTL). Nancy had not made much progress in this effort. She explained,
"In those days most poor people did not have a clue about how their bodies
worked. They thought birth control would inhibit their sexual functioning.
Women felt their man would not want them if they used birth control. It took
a lot of teaching and a lot of time to get someone to consent to birth control."

When Nancy arrived that day at her patient's small frame house, crowded
with children and stifling hot, she was horrified to hear the patient's account of

her delivery. Her son had been born en route to the university hospital where Nancy worked in a car her husband had borrowed. After the frightening birth, her husband rushed to the nearest hospital—a small community hospital where, because they had no money or insurance, she was refused admission. In fact, she was not even brought into the hospital. Rather, an emergency department (ED) staff member came to the car and, assured that the baby was OK and the mother was not bleeding profusely, sent her home. "At that time," said Nancy, "if you did not have money, you did not get care at these small hospitals."

Nancy examined the mother and her baby and, remarkably, found that they were both all right. She stayed for two hours, teaching the mother how to care for herself. Nancy arranged to stop by that evening when the husband would be home. With the mother's permission, Nancy would resume talking with him about birth control for his wife.

Nancy worked with the couple over several weeks. The husband resisted discussions of birth control. Nevertheless, Nancy tactfully persisted. She recalled, "I finally helped him see that having her tubes tied wouldn't have an impact on her sexuality. It took a lot of teaching. I had to educate him about basic anatomy. I also explained that he didn't have to tell his friends and that this would save her life. She kept saying to him, 'I'm tired.' When he finally agreed to a BTL, I felt I had participated in a real success story."

Nancy's efforts with this couple, however, were minor compared to the effort she had to make to gain acceptance by colleagues in the health departments where she was establishing pediatric clinics. She explained, "My job entailed setting up a systematic way to educate staff in local health departments to provide comprehensive pediatric, and later perinatal health care. I was trying to establish model clinics in the five county area. I was available to help upgrade services to children and later to pregnant women. Immediately it was clear that there was great resistance to working with an African-American person prepared at my level. Folks weren't ready to accept me. I would go to meetings as a colleague of the administrators and doctors from the university hospital, and the directors of the local health departments would single me out and say, 'I want to see your credentials.' Because the directors of the health departments had agreed with the university-based hospital that I could be there, I just moved ahead and tried to do my job."

Nancy continued, "It was rough at times. In one health department, one of the nurses would lock the examining room so that I could not use it. I just told the head nurse, 'If you want me to see patients, you will have to open the door to the examining room.' What kept me going was remembering the women I wanted to help."

The discrimination was not unfamiliar. Growing up the oldest of nine children in the 1940s in a rural, southern state, Nancy had sat in the back of the bus and used "Colored" bathrooms. She knew racism. She declared, "I was prepared for these people not to accept me, but I knew I had something to offer. I wanted to help the patients in these counties by getting these clinics up and running."

Nancy's persistence paid off. Eventually, she was accepted by the health department staff in one county—the poorest county in the state. "They had limited staff and they were desperate for help, so they didn't see my color so much," Nancy explained. She set about training the staff and developing the pediatric services, and very quickly she also established a pediatric and perinatal clinic. Delighted to have a "black doctor" in the health department, the patients started "coming out of the woodwork."

Nancy recalled, "These were patients who had never had prenatal care before because they did not feel they had a place to go. Before this clinic, prenatal care consisted of weighing people, taking their vital signs, and giving them a little bag of iron tablets. Soon our clinic offered physical examinations, lab work, nutritional counseling, Pap smears, and birth control counseling. We were giving real prenatal care. I had wonderful experiences with many, many women."

Nancy's reputation grew. The state began putting more money behind her efforts and eventually Nancy developed pediatric and prenatal clinics in all five target counties and, ultimately, in other counties as well. She said, "After our success in one county, my confidence increased. I went back to the counties where they hadn't wanted to work with me and said, 'Excuse me, but the state has sent me here to train you to do this. It is not a matter of whether you want this or not, because it's going to happen.'" Nancy continued, "By this time it was the early 80s and things were changing. Prejudice is learned, and while people couldn't change overnight, many could unlearn prejudice. Others retired, and as younger people came on the scene, things became different in regard to race. So I went from one county to another, setting up the clinics and training the nurses. Gradually they accepted me and my services."

After a number of years, 17 nurses, many of them nurse practitioners, were coordinating efforts in the pediatric and prenatal clinics throughout the state. Two of these nurses were African-American, like Nancy. Each coordinator was affiliated with a university-based hospital to ensure that staff would receive continuing education.

Throughout these years, Nancy continued to see countless patients, taking advantage of every opportunity to listen to their concerns and to teach them. "Women would come in for a postpartum visit. I would teach them about their bodies, encourage them to touch themselves and become familiar with their bodies. Most women did not understand birth control, for example, or associate the menstrual cycle with other physical symptoms. I would always tell them a little bit about something that I thought they could carry away with them."

Nancy reflected, "I could often pull an experience from my own past and use that to relate to the patient. I had been a teen mother, I had waited for hours in a free clinic and then been seen by a resident, medical student, or intern. I had been a smoker. I was not afraid to share these experiences with my patients because I wanted to help the patients. I can say to my patients, 'I know this is very hard. I have been poor. I know about these things.'"

Despite heavy administrative responsibilities, Nancy continues to see patients once a week. However, her primary job now is helping nurses in the clinics solve problems and provide excellent care. Recently a nurse called about a Hispanic patient who wanted to have a BTL after her delivery. In order for Medicaid to pay for the BTL, it had to occur during the short period of coverage for the delivery. Because the patient failed to bring the paperwork to the hospital when she delivered and could not communicate to the staff that she had completed the paperwork, she was sent home without the BTL. The nurse called Nancy to ask, "What can we do?" Nancy went to work. She reported, "It took about two hours, but I got the patient set up to come back in two days and have the BTL done. It was wonderful to be able to accomplish that. The nurse had confidence that I would help her, and I didn't want to let the nurse or the patient down. I usually get things done."

As the years have passed, Nancy has earned the respect of her nurse and physician colleagues. She observed, "My reputation with the people I work with is good. I've gone out and talked with these women to hear their concerns. I've tried to respond to their needs, and I've always been respectful of their values. Now they greet me with the greatest respect. What matters to me is how patients and people feel I have helped them; that is important to me. I have no wish for power, I just want to work with these women—to meet them where they are. And I feel I have done that. My work is deeply satisfying."

Enacting Artful Nursing

Nancy's personal experiences as a poor minority woman provided the primary basis for her life-long sense of identity with and compassion for this population. Her familiarity with the culture of the women and children she served provided a foundation for her vision for pediatric and perinatal clinics. Three features of community-based advocacy highlight the key nursing actions in Nancy's story.

- Commitment to advocacy
- Cultural competence
- Courage and advocacy

COMMITMENT TO ADVOCACY

An advocate is a person "who works with and on behalf of targeted individuals, assisting them in accessing needed resources" (McFarlane & Wiist, 1997, p. 239). This role is depicted in Nancy's sustained effort on behalf of poor African-American women. Motivated by her identification with these women, Nancy overcame political and personal obstacles to help poor women. "I have been poor. I know about these things," she declared. "What kept me going was remembering the women I wanted to help." This remembrance was key to her commitment to right the wrongs she herself had experienced from an unfeeling health care system. She knew what it was like to be overlooked, kept waiting for hours to see a health care provider, made to ride in the back of a bus, use "Colored" bathrooms, or feel held back by limited education. "I wanted to make it different for other young women," she explained.

Nancy's commitment was essential to her success as an advocate. This was true in part because the population-focused changes she sought were, like many population-focused advocacy efforts, infused with political, economic, and social factors as well as issues of power and control. Thus, advocating for this population was a slow, difficult, and challenging labor that required serious commitment. Such commitment is evident in the 25-year span of Nancy's story, during which her focus to help poor women in her state did not waver. Over the years, Nancy became educated, learned to navigate political and social systems, sustained her affiliation with poor women, and created satisfactory working relationships with resistant and racist colleagues in several public health departments. Undaunted by suspicious colleagues or locked examining rooms, she did not measure her value by the judgment of others, nor did their judgment diminish her commitment, without which it would have been impossible to realize her vision of the clinics.

Commitment was also necessary to sustain Nancy's efforts with patients. She worked with the values of the individuals she served. "I've gone out and talked with these women to hear their concerns. I've tried to respond to their needs and I've always been respectful of their values," she explained. Change was often slow. Because of a profound lack of knowledge, in many cases patients resisted becoming equal partners with Nancy in health-related issues. She worked for weeks and months to bring about acceptance of birth control or to teach women about their bodies. Nevertheless, Nancy was persistent. "I knew I had something to offer," she declared. "I wanted to help the patients in these counties by getting the pediatric clinics up and running." And as the patients came to her, she would "tell them a little bit about something that I thought they could carry away with them." Bit by bit she educated these women about their bodies and their babies. Eventually, after years of work and with functioning pediatric and prenatal clinics throughout the state, Nancy could conclude with great satisfaction, "I've gone out and done what felt right." Her commitment sustained her affiliation with the population she wanted to serve.

Underpinning her commitment was Nancy's ability to focus on the present. She dealt with each challenge as it arose, whether it was system wide or involved an individual patient. Further, she took great pleasure in the rewards of her work, declaring her winning efforts to get the young woman on birth control a "real success story." The gratitude of her patients, coupled with her sense of solidarity with these women, nourished over many years her larger efforts to make system-wide changes.

CULTURAL COMPETENCE

Nancy's commitment was to advocacy for poor women. To meet her goals, she had to achieve competence in a variety of cultures. Initially, she had to learn to navigate the culture of a university-based health care delivery system. Toward this end, she rose from an LPN to a master's prepared clinical nurse specialist with a focus in the health of women and children. She wrote a proposal outlining her goals. She recalled, "Somehow that little proposal got into the hands of someone at the university-based hospital where I was working," and soon she had an interview with the physicians who were to become her colleagues. Her proposal was funded, she was hired, and she moved into the culture of academic health care where she ultimately became a widely respected leader.

Nancy also needed to develop cultural competence in the arena of public health departments. This presented greater challenges given the racist nature of these settings in the early 1970s. While she supported the structure of public health departments that enabled access to health care for low-income individuals, the racist values of this culture excluded many patients of color. She could not accept this or discrimination, given her own values, which required her to "always be respectful to others."

There are limits to acculturation. For example, nurses are not expected to support culturally driven racism. Nancy recognized this, and despite her need for the cooperation of the public health department professionals, she refused to accept the racist culture of the system. She met head on the "great resistance to working with an African-American person prepared at my level," refusing to turn away from the social and political agendas driving the system. When locked out of an examining room, she explained, "If you want me to see patients, you will have to open the door to the examining room." Eventually her persistence paid off; she was accepted in the poorest county in the state, a county with limited staff, desperate for help, where they did not "see my color so much."

Once Nancy gained entry into one county and her skills in education and organization became evident, support for her efforts grew at the state level. Her reputation, persistence, and skill paid off: she was able to return with confidence and authority to the health departments that had previously rejected her with the words, "Excuse me, but the state has sent me here to train you to do this. It is not a matter of whether you want this or not, because it's going to happen."

Once she became a part of the health departments, Nancy worked within the system to make significant changes, teaching other practitioners how to address patients with respect and opening the doors to poor women who "came out of the woodwork" to see the "black doctor in the health department." In short, Nancy's cultural sensitivity and awareness enabled her to tolerate but not support an abhorrent racist culture, leading her to conclude that "prejudice is learned and can be unlearned," and ultimately enabling her to bring about significant needed change.

COURAGE AND ADVOCACY

Courage played a commanding role in Nancy's story. Acting on her conviction that "regardless of what color you are or how much money you have, health care should be equal," Nancy stood up for herself, for individual patients, and for groups of patients. Significantly, her courage arose from her desire to help others. "What kept me going was remembering the women I wanted to help," she explained.

The courage evident in Nancy's story was broad in scope. Faced with harsh colleagues who were not ready to "work with an African-American person prepared at my level," Nancy continued to show up despite their rude rejections and demands to "see your credentials." Yet throughout this trial of overt racism, Nancy avoided judgment, explaining that, "Prejudice is learned and while people couldn't change overnight, many could unlearn prejudiced behavior." Faced with rude rejection, Nancy "just moved ahead and tried to do my job . . . [and] gradually they accepted me and my service."

Nancy's response to resistant colleagues did not immediately translate into positive interactions. Armed with her commitment to the "women I wanted to help," she set about to change the status quo, and once she had the authority in the form of state support, she insisted that her work be tolerated. Recall her declaration to resistant colleagues: "It is not a matter of whether you want this or not, because it is going to happen." Courageously Nancy ploughed ahead, not losing sight of her goal. After years of effort, she could say with satisfaction, "My reputation with the people I work with is good. Now they greet me with the greatest respect. What matters to me is how patients and people feel I have helped them; that is important to me. I have no wish for power, I just want to work with these women—to meet them where they are. And I feel I have done that."

Challenges to Advocacy for Populations

Like all aspects of artful nursing, advocacy for populations may be met with constraints. They include the personal challenge of growth and change, the practical and conceptual concerns in nursing education related to community-based nursing, the challenges presented by entrenched political and social structures, and the assets and limitations of partnerships with communities.

Summing up her experience as a nurse working with inner-city African-Americans in the 1960s, Milio wrote, "It is dangerous to encourage people to talk—to express their feelings in words, to shape their ideas into coherent forms . . . everyone becomes more vulnerable, more exposed, and thus more equal" (1970, p. 191). Milio goes on to explain how in true partnerships out of which arise genuine dialogue, people may be frightened by their own feelings.

Everyone is changed and the process is ongoing, always calling for new change and response. She concludes, "The whole process [of genuine dialogue] is inherently dangerous. Only a belief in the human rightness of it, in its importance to human wholeness, makes it worth the effort" (p. 192).

Working to improve the lives of at-risk populations is indeed dangerous business that requires personal courage, persistence, and openness to growth and change. As Milio (1970) points out and Nancy's story corroborates, change is rarely easy. Further, advocacy for populations is slow, circuitous, and unpredictable. Cultural attitudes and perspectives of both the nurse and the population may be unconscious and outside awareness. What seems obvious in one culture may seem mysterious and illogical in another (Kemp, 1996). Respect for differences is key to confronting this aspect of population-focused advocacy. There are few structures in place to encourage true partnerships with disenfranchised populations. Political and social agendas must be skillfully navigated while the nurse develops awareness of cultural values and norms.

There are also constraints to working with populations at the most basic level of nursing education, where there is a lack of consistency with regard to teaching community health nursing (Drevdahl, 1995; Williams, 1997). Most students are taught community assessment with interventions directed toward individuals or families in the community rather than interventions to improve the health of a population or change the larger social structures that produce poor health. Further, the long-standing focus on caring for individuals in nursing education is sometimes taught at the expense of ignoring the concerns related to how one cares for communities (Chafey, 1997). This state of things in nursing education is in part a result of confusion within the profession over ideas and values. These include confusion about community-centered care versus individual- and family-centered care; health promotion versus treatment of illness; patient autonomy versus the good of the community, and the complexity and inherent difficulty of defining and implementing community interventions (Drevdahl, 1995).

Despite the fact that population-focused advocacy has been a part of the ideology of nursing since Wald's early efforts, nursing interventions designed to empower marginalized people and foster creative solutions to social and health problems continue to present great challenges. This is the case in part because of the complexity of working with groups of individuals, the time required to develop partnerships, and the social, political, and cultural barriers to cooperative endeavors (Drevdahl, 1995).

Relationships wherein there is genuine sharing of power are difficult to create and maintain (Drew, 1996; Milio, 1970). Indeed, it has been suggested that it may not be possible to have true collaborative and equal partnerships with populations given the differences in class, power, race, ethnicity, and education that often exist between the nurse and the target community (Drevdahl, 1995). However, it is possible to create a sense of reciprocity between nurses and communities whereby each learns from the other. Movement toward this end would be a large step.

Despite support within the nursing profession for community-based nursing, there is among some nurses a disregard for the broad social, political, and economic concerns that affect the health of marginalized populations. In a 1994 survey in which public health nurses were asked to identify important research questions related to public health, not one of 347 nurses identified questions of social or environmental factors (Misener, Watkins, & Ossege, 1994).

Not all nurses are cut out for the role so ably assumed by Nancy. However, while all nurses will not work directly with communities or specific populations, nurses can help shape political structures. For example, nurses can serve on city planning boards that make decisions related to economic growth and housing development. Nurses and nursing students can also examine their own role in supporting social structures that promote inequities, particularly in regard to health care. Further, nurses can become involved with communities through volunteering in community-focused activities like sheltered workshops, soup kitchens, or homeless shelters (Drevdahl, 1995). Students can try to arrange special projects for credit in which they work on a specific population-identified problem. Finally, from positions of involvement in communities, nurses can address issues of justice like the allocation of scarce resources and access to health care, identify populations that need services and involve them in planning and problem solving, and help shape just public policy (Chafey, 1997). Whatever the means, community involvement begins with an orientation toward community-based needs. Such an orientation represents a nursing perspective that extends beyond the individual nurse-patient relationship to shape one's work as a nurse.

Summary

The art of population-focused advocacy is honed over years of experience and requires commitment that can sustain the challenges inherent in working with diverse populations. Central to successful population-focused advocacy are cultural awareness, a posture of reciprocity, and an attitude of partnership with the community. Despite the constraints to population-focused advocacy, few areas in nursing offer such rich possibilities for making a positive and long-lasting impact upon the health of large numbers of individuals. Thus population-based advocacy is a deeply satisfying aspect of artful nursing.

References

Bent, K.N. (1999). The ecologies of community caring. *Advances in Nursing Science, 21*(14), 29–36.

Chafey, K. (1997). Caring is not enough: Ethical paradigms for community-based care. In B.W. Spradley & J.A. Allender (Eds.), *Readings in community health nursing* (pp. 211–220). Philadelphia, PA: Lippincott.

Drevdahl, D. (1995). Coming to voice: The power of emancipatory community interventions. *Advances in Nursing Science, 18*(20), 13–24.

Drew, J.C. (1996). Cultural competence in partnerships with communities. In E.T. Anderson & J.M. McFarlane (Eds.), *Community as partner* (pp. 138–157). Philadelphia, PA: Lippincott.

Fleck, L. (1991). Please don't tell. *Hastings Center Report,* November–December.

Gadow, S., & Schroeder, C. (1996). An advocacy approach to ethics and community health. In E.T. Anderson & J.M. McFarlane (Eds.), *Community as partner* (pp. 123–136). Philadelphia, PA: Lippincott.

Hitchcock, J.E., Schubert, P.E., & Thomas, S.A. (1999). *Community health nursing.* Boston, MA: Delmar Publishers.

Kang, R. (1995). Building community capacity for health promotion: A challenge for public health nurses. *Public Health Nursing, 12,* 312–318.

Kavanagh, K., Absalom, K., Beil, W., & Schliessmann, L. (1999). Connecting and becoming culturally competent: A Lakota example. *Advances in Nursing Science, 21*(3), 9–31.

Kemp, C. (1996). Refugee health and community nursing—Dallas, Texas. In E.T. Anderson & J.M. McFarlane (Eds.), *Community as partner* (pp. 360–374). Philadelphia, PA: Lippincott.

McFarlane, J., & Wiist, W. (1997). Preventing abuse to pregnant women: Implementation of a "mentormother" advocacy model. *Journal of Community Health Nursing, 14,* 237–249.

Milio, N. (1970). *9226 Kercheval.* Ann Arbor, MI: University of Michigan Press.

Misener, T.R., Watkins, J.G., & Ossege, J. (1994). Public health nursing research priorities: A collaborative Delphi study. *Public Health Nursing, 11*(2), 6674.

Spradley, B.W., & Allender, J.A. (1997). *Readings in community health nursing.* Philadelphia, PA: Lippincott.

Thomas, S.A. (1999). Caring in community health nursing. In J.E.Hitchcock, P.E. Schubert, & S.A. Thomas (Eds.), *Community health nursing* (pp. 3–16). Boston, MA: Delmar Publishers.

Wald, L. (1971). *The house on Henry Street.* New York, NY: Dover Publications (original work published 1915).

Williams, C.A. (1997). Community health nursing—What is it? In B.W. Spradley & J.A. Allender (Eds.), *Readings in community health nursing* (pp. 101–109). Philadelphia, PA: Lippincott.

Willis, E.M., Biggins, A.L., & Donovan, J.E. (1999). In J.E. Hitchcock, P.E. Schubert, & S.A. Thomas (Eds.), *Community health nursing* (pp. 209–224). Boston, MA: Delmar Publishers.

APPLICATION

....

ACTIVITY I
Group Discussion: Analysis of the Story

1. Discuss the traits evident in Nancy's story that led to her success as a community-focused advocate.

2. Describe disenfranchised population groups within your own community. What have you learned from Nancy's story that would help you go about working with these groups as a community-focused nurse advocate?

3. What do you imagine you would have done if you had been locked out of an examining room because of racist beliefs about you?

ACTIVITY II
Case Analysis and Group Discussion: Understanding Different Perspectives

This is a case with compelling ethical challenges. However, you are *not* to focus only on "what is the right thing to do." Your job is to try to *understand* the patient's perspective and the perspective of the patient's sister, to examine your own biases for and against the patient and his sister, and to try to see *both* perspectives in this complex case. Try not to get distracted by the ethical question of what the nurse or doctor should do in this situation.

> Arturo was a 21-year-old Hispanic male who, as a result of gang violence, sustained a gunshot wound to his abdomen. He had no insurance. Medicaid was paying his bills. He was hospitalized and treated for the gunshot wound. He was discharged after a short hospital stay to complete his recovery at home. Arturo told his nurse practitioner he was HIV-positive, and this was confirmed by serology. When Arturo was discharged, the nurse practitioner recommended a daily home nursing visit for his wound care. However, Medicaid will not fund a nursing visit if a caregiver lives in the home who can provide care for the patient. Maria, the patient's sister, lived

in the home and was willing to accept the burden of the daily wound care and dressing changes.

Maria had been like a mother to Arturo since their mother had died ten years earlier. Arturo did not mind if Maria provided his care, but he was insistent that she was not to be told of his HIV-positive status. He had always been on good terms with Maria, but she did not know he was actively homosexual. Arturo did not want her to know this, and his greatest fear was that his father might find out he was homosexual, since his father looked upon homosexuality with great disdain.

Maria's decision to accept responsibility for the dressing changes was difficult for her. She had only recently completed her GED and had been given a scholarship to attend a community college for two years. Because of transportation complications, she could not attend school and do the dressing changes; hence her agreement to provide care to her brother meant she would have to refuse the scholarship. She agreed to accept the responsibility for her brother's care and turn down the scholarship since "he is my brother and has no one else."

Aspects of this case have been adapted from Fleck, L. (1991). Please don't tell. *Hastings Center Report,* November–December.

GROUP DISCUSSION QUESTIONS

1. What are the main concerns of this patient? Include a discussion of his physical, emotional, and relationship concerns. Consider also the patient's race, social class, income, health, and family situation and how they inform his concerns.

2. Does the patient reflect any stereotypes in our culture? Are his concerns "typical" of someone who falls into these stereotypes?

3. What are the main concerns of the sister? Include a discussion of her physical, emotional, and relationship concerns. Consider also her race, social class, income, health, and family situation and how they inform her concerns.

4. Now consider your own concerns in working with this family. Discuss any conflicts you might feel.

5. For whom do you feel the most compassion, Arturo or Maria? What from your own experience makes it difficult to feel compassion for either of these

characters? What from your own life experiences make it easy to feel compassion for either of these characters?

6. What are the aspects of this case that cause you to have difficulty seeing Arturo or Maria's perspective?

7. Do all the students in your group share similar feelings about Arturo and Maria? How do the responses in your group differ?

ACTIVITY III
Self-Reflection: Examining One's Own Biases

Write your responses to the following questions, based on the case presented and the group discussion:

1. In the first paragraph, give an overview of any biases you identified that you have or that society has toward the patient. Be specific as you describe these biases.

2. In a second paragraph, analyze these biases by putting yourself in the shoes of the patient or the group represented by this patient. What might his concerns be related to social biases?

3. In a final paragraph try to relate the experience of identifying and analyzing your and society's biases to your future role as a nurse. For example, are you more sympathetic toward one or the other of these persons? How might your response to the patient change if you look at the situation from the perspective of the sister? How might your biases affect your delivery of good nursing care?

ACTIVITY IV
Group Activity: Learning from Each Other

1. Work in pairs with one other member of your group. If possible, select someone you do not know well.

2. Identify one difference between you. This might take some time, but stay with it until you identify one real difference. This might be related to religious or spiritual orientation, beliefs about healthy behaviors including smoking or drinking, beliefs about a controversial issue like abortion or sexual orientation, or your opinions about a value in nursing, or a political issue.

3. Taking turns, your task in the next 15 to 20 minutes is to explain your position in regard to your differences to your partner, with the intent of helping your partner understand that position. The role of the listener is to try to understand, asking questions as necessary but not interrupting.

4. At the conclusion of this activity, discuss your experience. What were the challenges to listening carefully to a position that differed from your own? Were you able to listen with an open mind? If so, what facilitated your ability to hear what your partner was saying? What made this difficult?

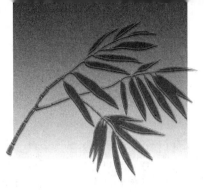

CHAPTER 7

Supporting Spirituality

....

Introduction

Noted scientist Stephen J. Gould maintains that science and spiritual concerns, the two great tools of human understanding, operate in complementary (not contrary) fashion (1999). According to Gould, scientific and spiritual matters should be "equal, mutually respecting partners, each the master of its own domain" (p. 59).

Nurses depend on science, with its focus on the factual state of the natural world, to guide patient care and treatment decisions. In complementary fashion, nurses rely on knowledge of the spiritual to guide their responses to patient questions of meaning and purpose.

Spirituality is most clearly manifested in situations that move one by their beauty, clarity, pain, or joy (Brussat & Brussat, 1996). Spiritual experiences may involve a heightened feeling of connection to another person, to a higher being, or to the whole of life or an increased sensitivity to the pain and suffering that touch every life. People respond spiritually to religious rituals; the beauty of nature; deeply felt moments shared with others; music, poetry, or visual arts; memories of loved persons who have died; stories of liberation or oppression; or their reflections on the meaning of life, suffering, forgiveness, or any human experience.

In her treatise on the spiritual life, written in 1860 and recently republished, Florence Nightingale ascribed to spirituality those "feelings called forth by the consciousness of a presence of higher nature than human, unconnected with the material" (Calabria & Macrae, 1994, p. 120). In recent years there has been renewed attention to the spiritual care of patients (Laukhuf & Werner, 1998; Wright, 1998). Indeed, in *Nursing: Human Science and Human Care* (1985), Watson defines nursing as a "human-to-human care process with spiritual dimensions" (p. 37). Further, the International Council of Nurses (ICN) Code for Nurses states, "The nurse, in providing care, promotes an environment in which the values, customs and spiritual beliefs of the individual are respected" (1973, p. 465).

While most nurses have encountered patient suffering and have observed patients' struggle for meaning, many fail to recognize and address the patient's spiritual concerns (Sumner, 1998; Wright, 1998). Others take a restricted perspective on the dimension of spirituality, failing to recognize expressions of spirituality (Khan & Steeves, 1994).

This chapter examines three aspects of spirituality that may guide recognition and response to the patient's spiritual needs.
- Spirituality and religion
- Manifestations of spirituality
- Spiritual care

Spirituality and Religion

Though she was a member of the Church of England, Florence Nightingale showed little interest in conventional religion. Rather, she believed that all things in creation were rooted in the same spiritual reality and shared the same inner divinity. Nightingale believed that this inner divinity was a part of human nature and the purpose of human life was the unfolding of inner divinity. In 1860 she wrote, "The eternal source of truth, of goodness, and wisdom is ever ready to supply the faculties of mankind with means of increase, so that to-day may always be richer than yesterday, if these means are taken" (Calabria & Macrae, 1994, p. 119). According to Nightingale, one role of the nurse was to help create an environment in which "the unfolding of inner divinity" could occur (Macrae, 1995).

The distinction that Nightingale made between spirituality (expressed for Nightingale as mysticism) and religion (practices of the Church of England) is often missed by contemporary nurses. Indeed, many nurses equate spirituality and religion (Halstead & Mickley, 1997; Mayer, 1992; Ross, 1994). Furthermore, many nurses recognize spirituality only if it fits with their own religious framework. This is a shortsighted, narrow, and perilous position that limits recognition of the spirituality of a patient who may not be religious or whose religious practices are unfamiliar to the nurse; it may prevent the nurse from responding to the totality of the patient's experience.

What then are the distinctions between spirituality and religion? Spirituality is broadly concerned with questions of meaning and purpose; the need for hope and creative expression; familiar rituals and meaningful work; and relationships to self, others, the natural order, or a higher power (Clark, 1997; Halstead & Mickley, 1997; Wright, 1998). Spirituality represents striving "to actualize the real self" (Watson, 1985, p. 57) and is "a dimension of the human spirit which, connected to a larger 'something'—be it God, the Universe, Nature or Community—transcends the everyday [physical] world" (Kahn & Steeves, 1994).

Religion refers to "codified beliefs about the meaning of the universe and its expression in myths and practices" (Taylor, Amenta, & Highfield, 1995, p. 32). While many formal religions address spiritual concerns, spirituality goes beyond religion, escaping the confines of churches, synagogues, and temples (Sumner, 1998). Thus a patient who has no religious affiliation may have a well-developed sense of the spiritual.

The failure of many nurses to recognize patients' spirituality apart from religious beliefs stems from the vagueness about what constitutes spirituality. Religions can be defined by codes, practices, rituals, and tenets; spirituality cannot. While spirituality is expressed uniquely by each individual, there are nevertheless certain shared features of spirituality that can help the nurse recognize the spiritual needs of patients.

Manifestations of Spirituality

In Alice Walker's novel *The Color Purple* (1982), Shug says to her friend: "God love[s] everything you love—and a mess of stuff you don't. But more than anything else, God love[s] admiration. . . . I think it pisses God off if you walk by the color purple in a field somewhere and don't notice it" (p. 167). Shug is suggesting that the beauty of the color purple in a field is an expression of God. While Shug was reminded of God in a purple flower, others might be reminded of the spiritual upon hearing beautiful music, or seeing a sunset, or watching a child play. Attentiveness is required to appreciate expressions of spirituality; some are easy to see while others are as unexpected and easy to overlook as a purple flower in a field. Inattentive, Shug would have missed the flower.

Like everyone else, patients have spiritual concerns. Indeed, these concerns are often provoked by intense experiences such as illness or dying. It has been suggested that "journeys of the soul and adventures in change often begin unhappily, born of pain, disappointment, or shock. When we're suffering . . . we feel things more acutely" (Katz, 1999, p. 15). And in fact, terminally ill adults demonstrate a greater concern with spirituality than other groups of adults (Kahn & Steeves, 1994).

Patients' spiritual experiences may reflect a sense of connection to or alienation from self, others, or a higher being (Burkhardt, 1994). Spiritual themes are expressed in comments about the meaning or purpose in life, or guilt or anxiety about unreconciled relationships; remarks about fulfilling relationships or reconciliation; statements about the future including changes in one's sense of self; observations about the positive or negative impact of illness on relationships, work, or family; challenges to or confirmation of patient beliefs or values; comments that indicate the patient has made a "deal" with God; and feelings of grief, hopelessness, helplessness, despair as well as joy, gratitude, peace, hope, and acceptance (Clark, 1997; Laukhuf & Werner, 1998; Taylor et al., 1995).

Patients may indicate spiritual concerns with comments such as "I'm scared," "Please help me," "I feel so alone," "I am ready to die," "I do not want to leave my family," "I am peaceful," or "No more, I've had enough." Sometimes patients refer to their religious beliefs or faith in a God with comments like "Why did God do this to me?" "I've always been religious, I don't see why I should be punished like this," or "God will take care of me," and "I am ready to go and be with God." Still other patients indicate their spiritual state through nonverbal behaviors including withdrawal, crying, anger, restlessness, inability to cope, and peacefulness (Taylor et al., 1995).

Not all indicators of spirituality reflect spiritual need; many highlight the spiritual assets and strengths of patients. Further, many patients may not recognize as spiritual their own expressions of spirituality, and in some situations, patients may not wish to share their spiritual experiences with the nurse. In these cases, it is important to respect the patient's privacy and be a silent and compassionate witness to the patient's experience without trying to give words to it.

Spiritual Care

In recent years, a number of researchers have found a positive relationship between spirituality and the patient's sense of well-being (Kahn & Steeves, 1994). For example, a study of 30 newly diagnosed cancer patients found that faith, broadly understood as a connection to God, was a major factor in patients' ability to cope. Interestingly, 87 percent of these patients stated that religion, particularly church attendance, was not central to their lives (O'Conner, Wicker, & Germino, 1990).

Like expressions of spirituality, spiritual care must be unique and fit the situation. Spiritual care turns on the nurse's spiritual awareness and receptivity to the unknown and on an openness on the part of the nurse and patient (Stiles, 1994). The essence of spiritual care is not religious doctrine or dogma but "the fundamental human capacity to enter into the world of others and respond with feeling. It requires from the patient and the nurse a willingness to share pain and suffering, with all the ambiguity, messiness, and risk inherent in such an undertaking" (Mayer, 1992, p. 51). The goals of spiritual care are to honor the patient's expressions of spirituality, support beliefs and rituals (Laukhuf & Werner, 1998), and relieve the alienation of patients who are struggling with questions of meaning (Younger, 1995).

One way to think about spiritual care is to think about what the nurse does *not* do. Since spirituality must be defined for oneself and cannot be taught or bestowed on others, the nurse must resist the temptation to define spiritual truth for the patient (Mayer, 1992). Statements like "God loves you" or "God doesn't send us more than we can bear" may ring true for the nurse, but they may be offensive to patients with different beliefs and thus may serve to silence patients, increasing feelings of alienation and loneliness. Nor is it useful to apply a problem-solving approach to spiritual matters. Neither the nurse nor the chaplain can deliver answers to a patient or resolve a patient's spiritual concerns since "spiritual qualities are not given but achieved . . . [and] answers to fundamental questions can't be given but [are] discovered" (Mayer, 1992, p. 34).

The appropriate nursing role is to help with the process of discovery, not try to deliver a neatly packaged answer. Recall how Elizabeth in Chapter 4 recognized that she could not "fix" Leah's deep grief. Her recognition spared Leah an intrusive effort to make things right while providing her the comfort of having someone with her. Leah remained deeply sad, but she was not alone in her grief. Similarily, David, in Chapter 3, came to understand Lois's grief and tried to find how he might best help her. The outcome would have been different had David silenced Lois with words like, "Chip is dead. This is God's will. You must accept it."

Nurses do sometimes talk about religious beliefs or spiritual matters with patients. Indeed, such conversations, including acknowledgment of shared beliefs, are frequently appropriate and can be useful to both patient and nurse. However, the nurse must avoid forcing beliefs, answers, or even conversations about spirituality upon the patient. In matters of spirituality, the patient leads. Imposition of the nurse's beliefs or solutions onto the patient is deeply offensive because spirituality is a unique expression of the individual.

Spiritual care includes all the features of caring depicted in Chapter 4, in addition to an awareness of the spiritual. Spiritual care does not involve specific interventions such as turning a patient to prevent skin breakdown but colors the whole of the nurse's response to the patient. At its best, spiritual care results in a shared experience that is affirming to the nurse and the patient. For example, the nurse may feel the same sense of peace as the family when a loved one dies (Stiles, 1994). Aspects of spiritual care that have been identified by patients include the use of humor, telling the truth, managing pain, offering comfort through touch, and spending time explaining, teaching, and preparing patients and family members for the experience of dying (Stiles, 1994).

Spiritual care may also entail arranging for familiar rites like communion, praying, setting up an altar, or reading from sacred texts. If the patient desires, the nurse can call the chaplain or the patient's spiritual mentor. One nurse working in oncology reported how, at a dying patient's request, she and the chaplain arranged for the patient to be baptized in the Hubbard tank used to debried burn patients. While it is quicker and often easier to give an answer than to be present for a patient grappling with matters of the spirit, the nurse needs to remember that easy answers silence the patient, as do quick reassurances. As Elizabeth demonstrated in her care of Leah (Chapter 4), sometimes all the nurse can do is quietly hold the patient.

The story that follows depicts the dying of Mr. Warren, a spiritual man who also was religious. Unlike those patients for whom religion offers little or no comfort, Mr. Warren's peaceful death was enabled by his religious beliefs and his spiritual practice.

Gwyn's Story

Mr. Warren was a successful businessman who was widely respected in his native southern state. Throughout his life, he had devoted much of his time to religious causes and to helping others. During the tumultuous sixties when the Civil Rights Movement was gaining momentum, he led his local church and the community toward a peaceful integration of the public schools. He traveled widely in support of the numerous Christian missions he had helped establish throughout the world.

At the age of 78, Mr. Warren, who had always been healthy and fit, developed unrelenting and severe gastric distress. Despite a bland diet and medications, his pain persisted for weeks. Eventually, the pain increased to such an extent that Mr. Warren was admitted to the hospital for diagnostic studies. The news was not good—Mr. Warren had aggressive pancreatic cancer. He was transferred to the oncology unit to be worked up for treatment. Gwyn became his primary nurse.

"His cancer was extremely aggressive. He lost ground very quickly. Two days after his admission he was obstructed and we had to put in a nasogastric tube," Gwyn explained.

Initially Mr. Warren expressed a wish for aggressive treatment. A plan was made to fly him to a regional medical center to undergo extensive and somewhat experimental surgery. After surgery he would return to the local hospital for follow-up treatment. The company for which he had worked offered their jet for the trip. Ready to travel, Mr. Warren underwent one final test, which revealed that the cancer had permeated his abdominal cavity. Aggressive surgery would be futile. The trip was canceled.

Gwyn observed, "Mr. Warren must have been intensely let down to hear this news, but he never expressed his feelings aloud. Well informed, he knew the hopelessness of his situation, but he accepted the sudden news of his terminal illness without protest."

Mr. and Mrs. Warren, married for 48 years, had five adult children. Upon hearing of their father's illness, the children arrived from various parts of the country to be with their parents. Upset and fearful for their father and concerned for their mother, they took turns being with their parents in the small hospital room. The family would gather twice each day, expectantly awaiting the report from the physician. As the first week of Mr. Warren's illness unfolded, there was little good news. Mr. Warren rapidly grew weaker. Gwyn recalled, "My role during the first week of his illness was primarily to educate the patient and family regarding the tests he was undergoing and then to support them through the trauma of the diagnosis and the news of aggressive and extensive nature of his cancer. His care was not complex, so I incorporated his children into his care by showing them how to help him walk in the halls and to do his mouth care."

In the second week of his hospitalization, palliative surgery was proposed to remove some of the cancer and insert a gastrostomy tube through the abdominal wall to drain the stomach contents, thus enabling them to remove the nasogastric tube. The surgeon's report brought more bad news. Mr. Warren's abdomen was so studded with cancer that he could not even insert the gastrostomy tube. Not only was there no treatment for Mr. Warren, but he would also have to endure the discomfort of the nasogastric tube until he died. "Things were happening quickly for this patient and his family," Gwyn observed.

Following his surgery, the family established a daily routine around Mr. Warren's needs. Mrs. Warren and the children came early in the morning to see the physician when he made rounds. While Mrs. Warren was reluctant to help directly with her husband's care, the children shaved their father, helped him ambulate or sit in a chair, and did his mouth care. His wife read the Bible to him. At day's end everyone left except one of his children, who would sit quietly with him until a private duty nurse arrived for the night shift.

Gwyn observed, "I was struck by his willingness to be cared for, his grace in giving up his abilities to meet his own bodily needs. For almost 50 years he had provided for his family, and now they were providing for him. He accepted their care with gratitude rather than apology or resistance."

By the end of the second week of his illness, everyone including Mr. Warren knew that he was dying. While he did not speak directly of his death, he acknowledged it indirectly in several ways. For example, after his surgery, he arranged meetings with several individuals to finalize business-related concerns. He asked his children to select a plot under a tree for his burial and to pick out a casket. He offered words of reassurance to his family, telling his wife, "It's not your time to go; you will be OK until your time comes" and telling his children: "We all have to go sometime, and something has to take us. I am peaceful."

Gwyn reflected, "The family was right there for Mr. Warren and he was there for them. My role was to keep him clean, turned, and comfortable and to answer the family's questions. I also did some family teaching, helping them know what they might expect as his dying unfolded. I don't know whether it was their support and love that was key, but I never saw him in the least bit upset or anxious. I have never had a patient with a nasogastric tube who didn't complain a little—they are so unpleasant; yet he never once complained about anything." Gwyn concluded, "I was intrigued by the quiet and deliberate way he was dealing with his death. I was learning a great deal from Mr. Warren about acceptance and facing death without any evidence of fear."

Ten days after his diagnosis, it became apparent that Mr. Warren's kidneys were failing. Initially, no one approached Mr. Warren about treatment options. His children were divided in their opinions—some favored dialysis but others opposed any treatment that would prolong his dying. Conflicted, his wife turned to Gwyn, "What should we do? I cannot imagine how I can survive without him, my life is so closely a part of his. I do not want him to suffer, but I cannot just let him go."

Gwyn observed, "My one regret about caring for Mr. Warren was that I failed his wife at this point. I should have offered her information and listened to her concerns. But instead of hearing her out and giving her the benefit of my experience, I suggested she talk to the doctor. I was so busy that day, I felt I couldn't take the time she needed. While I didn't have any answers for her, I know she needed what we all need—someone to be there in our struggles and uncertainties and our fears. She was far less accepting of the situation than her husband. So I failed Mrs. Warren—and myself—by passing up an opportunity to be with her as she worked through the question of whether to begin dialysis."

By the next day Mr. and Mrs. Warren had spoken with the physician about treatment options. Given his poor prognosis, Mr. Warren decided not to undergo dialysis. "It's time for me to go," he concluded and reassuring his family he said, "Things are not going well for me physically, but otherwise, it is all going very well."

As his renal failure progressed, Mr. Warren could no longer walk in the halls or tolerate sitting in a chair. His children continued to help by shaving him, providing mouth care, and washing his face. His periods of mental clarity were diminishing. He was often confused and mostly slept, rousing only when the family spoke to him. Gwyn told the family that he would probably die within the next several days.

The day of his death began uneventfully; the family met the doctor for his rounds and then began their customary vigil at his bedside. Midmorning, his breathing suddenly became irregular and shallow, and he did not respond at all to the family gathered in his room. Gwyn told them, "I think he will die soon." Mrs. Warren, positioned in a chair next to his bed, quietly wept.

As Gwyn was preparing to leave for the day, she assessed Mr. Warren one last time for pain. He was resting peacefully and in no apparent distress. She told the family she would be leaving soon but would like to join them before she went home. The family welcomed Gwyn. Returning shortly, she stood quietly for a few minutes near the door, knowing that she had come back to say good-bye to her patient.

Suddenly Gwyn was astonished to hear Mr. Warren say in a remarkably strong voice, "The Lord has blessed us in so many ways. He will provide an answer." Then he was quiet.

"I was stunned by the strength of his voice and his clarity," Gwyn stated. "He had spoken little for several days, and most of what he had said reflected his confusion secondary to progressive renal failure. Now he was speaking in a clear, strong voice."

Throughout the next hour, Mr. Warren spoke intermittently about going home and his wish to say good-bye. He told his family he was ready to go, and at one point directly asked, "Do you want me to go home now?"

Gwyn encouraged the tearful family, "Tell him it is OK for him to go. Tell him you will be OK."

Individually each one spoke, "Do whatever is most peaceful for you. We are all OK. Go on home."

As Mrs. Warren said her good-byes, she lingered over her husband with her cheek against his as she wept and whispered, "I'll be OK, I'll be OK."

Gwyn remembered thinking, "It was like she was trying to convince him as well as herself that she would be OK. She did not want to let her husband go, she was not at all clear that she would be OK, but she wanted to release him to his death. I felt badly for her, because she could not imagine her life without her husband."

Mr. Warren was quiet for a short while and then suddenly said, "I need to stand up. I haven't been on my feet in a week and I may faint. You will have to help me, I need to stand up so I can leave."

A daughter replied, "Daddy, you don't need to walk where you are going."

Smiling in recognition, Mr. Warren said, "Oh, yes, you are right."

Minutes later he said, "Show me the exit. Can I go now?"

Another daughter replied, "You know the way. You are showing us."

Gwyn watched and listened, remaining apart from the family near the door to her patient's room. "They were all participating in his dying. The only thing I did for them was to encourage them to talk to him and provide the quiet and privacy they needed. At one point the oncologist came by. I signaled to him to be quiet. He stood by the bed for a few minutes, not speaking. I, too, stood by quietly, watching this remarkable dying. I remember thinking, I can't believe this. He is inviting them to go with him as far as they can go. I was overwhelmed and moved by what I was witnessing."

At one point Mr. Warren said, "I need to sit up so you can pray for me and I can go on home."

A family member suggested they say the Lord's prayer and started with the words, "Our Father who art in heaven."

In a surprisingly strong voice Mr. Warren interrupted, "No, you repeat the prayer after me. I will lead you."

And line by line Mr. Warren led his grieving family in the Lord's prayer, closing with the words, "Thank you, Lord, for the good experiences of this day. For Christ's sake, Amen."

Mr. Warren died a few hours later.

Ten years after his death, Gwyn closed her story with a tribute to her patient, "At the time I had no idea how I would be changed by this experience. It was not an immediate change, but it provoked my interest in spirituality. I had grown up in a church but had rejected formal religions. I had given no thought to spiritual or religious matters for many years. After Mr. Warren's death, I found myself drawn to books and conversations about spirituality. I continue on what I call a spiritual quest. I have more questions than answers, but I have a new awareness of the spiritual aspect of life. I owe that to Mr. Warren, and I am deeply grateful to him."

Enacting Artful Nursing

This story depicts the death of an individual who was sensitive to spiritual matters and who was also religious. The comfort of religious beliefs and practices provided the framework for Mr. Warren's peaceful dying. Many patients do not experience this kind of comfort and, indeed, some individuals are deeply spiritual but do not take part in formal religion. Others, like Mrs. Warren, may observe formal religious practices but find a lack of comfort in them at the time of great loss. Artful nursing includes respecting expressions of the human spirit, regardless of whether or not they are manifest through formal religious frameworks, and regardless of whether their expression is one of peaceful acceptance, questioning, or agony.

Three key nursing actions that guide the nursing response are:

- The search for meaning
- Spiritual sensitivity
- Supporting spirituality

THE SEARCH FOR MEANING

Physician Oliver Sacks (1984) described the poignant and individual nature of the struggle to find meaning during his slow recovery from a serious fracture of his leg. Despite the physician's declaration that there was "nothing wrong" with his leg, Sacks was unable to feel or move his leg during the early weeks of his recovery. Powerless to resume walking, Sacks described a time of deep spiritual agony wherein he could do nothing but wait for understanding: "A sense of utter hopelessness swept over me. I felt myself sinking. The abyss engulfed me. . . . I had to be still, and wait in the darkness, to feel it as holy, the darkness of God, and not simply as blindness and bereftness (though it entailed, indeed, total blindness and bereftness). I had to acquiesce, even be glad, that my reason was confounded and that my powers and faculties had no locus of action and could not be exerted to alter my state. I had not sought this, but it had happened, and so I should accept it—accept this strange passivity and night . . . not with anger, not with terror, but with gratitude and gladness (pp. 109, 112).

The search for meaning, depicted by Sacks as a paradoxical passage, is common among patients whose lives or routines are threatened by illness. For many this entails a visible struggle wherein, as Sacks says, one feels engulfed by an abyss. This was evident in Mrs. Warren's lament that she could not imagine herself without her husband. For others, like Mr. Warren, there is little outward evidence of struggle though it is unlikely that Mr. Warren had arrived at this point without experiencing some grief. Regardless of the forms of patient concerns about meaning, these are spiritual concerns, and the nurse's recognition of the patient's search for meaning is the starting point for spiritual care.

For Mr. Warren, the meaning of his life and death was entwined with his views of family roles and relationships. As family provider, he took care of incomplete business-related concerns, imparted comfort to his family, and close to death, resumed his role as head of the family to lead the Lord's prayer. At the same time, understanding that he was a beloved husband and father, he gratefully accepted the love and support of his family and the comfort of their presence.

Mr. Warren's peaceful dying was also framed by his religious beliefs. He viewed his death as "going home" and recognized with a smile that he did not need to "walk where he was going." Confident in his beliefs, he stated: "The Lord has blest us in so many ways. He will provide an answer." Indeed, his religious beliefs so structured his dying that his last words expressed his gratitude: "Thank you Lord for the good experiences of this day."

Less peaceful, Mrs. Warren raised questions about meaning as she recognized that her husband was dying. Having been married for almost 50 years, she was unable to imagine her life without her husband, acknowledging that her life was "a part of his." His death meant a part of her would die, and thus she grappled with her fears and his need to have a peaceful death, uncomplicated by futile treatments.

While Mr. Warren's family relationships and religious beliefs provided a framework for a peaceful death, this is not the case for all individuals. In *A Lesson Before Dying* (Gaines, 1993), Jefferson, a young black man living in the South in the 1950s, was falsely convicted of murder and sentenced to die. His godmother asked a young black teacher, Grant, to talk with Jefferson over the weeks before his death to help him "die like a man." Reluctantly, Grant took up the challenge, visiting Jefferson in jail several times a week. Jefferson remained defeated, fearful, angry, and indifferent to Grant's presence. As the date of Jefferson's execution approached, Grant challenged him with the words, "White people believe that they're better than anyone else on earth. . . . The last thing they ever want is to see a Black man stand, and think, and show that common humanity that is in us all. It would destroy their myth . . . as long as none of us stand, they're safe" (p. 192). Upon hearing Grant's words, Jefferson began to see the possibility of facing his executioners with dignity by walking "tall and straight" to his death. Confronting the legacy of white supremacy, Jefferson shifted from a defeated boy into "the strongest man in that crowded [execution] room" (p. 253). This radical movement, while not denying the tragedy of Jefferson's death, brought meaning to his dying.

Like Jefferson, many individuals search for meaning when faced with grave illness and death. Not everyone finds comfort and peace as readily as Mr. Warren. For some the search is difficult, a descent into darkness and agony. Some patients die alone without friends or family. Others have no religious beliefs, or they find little comfort in familiar religious frameworks. Questions of meaning are often couched in experiences in which the patient, like Sacks, must wait for understanding in the darkness, engulfed by a "sense of abomination and despair, a sense of a hideous and unspeakable hell" (Sacks, 1984, p. 112).

The search for meaning is deeply personal; hence no one, including the nurse, can show a patient the way out of the darkness of grief and loss. Only Mrs. Warren could bring new meaning to her life as it was redefined by her husband's death. In turn, only Mr. Warren could reach a peaceful acceptance of his death. However, the nurse can make a fundamental difference in the spiritual experience of the patient. While spiritual struggles like Mrs. Warren's search for meaning stand on their own and do not require interpretation by the nurse or an easy fix, they do require attention, a valued expression of spiritual care. Gwyn recognized this in acknowledging that Mrs. Warren did not need answers, but "she needed what we all need—someone to be there in our struggles and uncertainties and our fears." Had Gwyn responded to Mrs. Warren with a statement like "It is so hard to lose someone you love" or "I don't have the answer, but I will be with you as you try to understand what is happening," she might have broken Mrs. Warren's isolation in her effort to make sense of the loss of her husband.

It is not easy for the nurse to be with someone whose agony and pain are spiritual and cannot be relieved by medication or a well-developed nursing care plan. It is much easier to be with patients like Mr. Warren, who do not voice questions about meaning. Notably, Gwyn turned away from Mrs. Warren's explicit plea, "What should we do?" and her lament: "I cannot imagine how I can survive without him, my life is so closely a part of his . . . I cannot just let him go." Gwyn justified her choice not to be present to Mrs. Warren by the genuine claim that other demands required her attention. However, it should be noted that Gwyn was so intrigued by Mr. Warren's peaceful acceptance of his death that she returned to his room after her shift was complete to say good-bye and remained until he died. This was not her response to Mrs. Warren's plea.

Critical to the capacity to be with a patient like Mrs. Warren, whose struggle for meaning was dark and difficult, is the acceptance by the nurse of her own darkness and fears and the acknowledgment that true questions of meaning are shared by all humanity (Younger, 1995). By accepting our own darkness and fear, we join the human experience fully. Had Gwyn recognized this, she could have responded to Mrs. Warren from her own experience of spiritual struggle, thereby tempering the isolation and agony of her loss and spiritual pain.

SPIRITUAL SENSITIVITY

Depicting his friendship with a young medical student who was tormented by his addiction to cocaine, physician Verghese (1998) described the dynamic of illness for the human spirit: "It is a terrifying experience [to be ill]. It's important that you realize that every illness, whether it's a broken bone or a bad pneumonia, comes with a spiritual violation that parallels the physical ailment" (p. 98). Verghese suggests that the experience of illness disrupts the body while also provoking questions like Why me? and How will I manage this experience?

Mr. Warren gave no indication of spiritual violation accompanying his illness. Understanding himself as a religious and spiritual man, he quietly embraced his dying in the recognition that he was "going home." The spiritual violation in Gwyn's story was most evident in the impact of Mr. Warren's illness on his wife. Mrs. Warren, conflicted over whether to support dialysis, struggled in the face of her fears of a life without her husband.

Gwyn's ability to honor Mr. Warren and his family's spiritual experience turned on a sensitivity that allowed her to notice and appreciate religious orientations that were different from her own. Her sensitivity to spiritual matters was not tied to religious beliefs shared with Mr. Warren or his family, or even to an explicit consciousness of spiritual matters. Gwyn had given no thought to spiritual or religious themes for many years. Her ability to respond sensitively to spiritual concerns grew out of the fact that she felt connected to her patients as fellow humans. What mattered to the patient mattered to Gwyn, whether in her own mind she called it spiritual, suffering, loneliness, or pain control. This was evident in her lament when she failed to respond with compassion to Mrs. Warren: "I failed myself and Mrs. Warren." Gwyn's eagerness to see Mr. Warren each day, her incorporation of the family into his care, her respectful presence as he was dying, and her gratitude to him for awakening her own spiritual quest were all stimulated by her recognition of herself as kin to her patient.

SUPPORTING SPIRITUALITY

In many cases, supporting the patient's expressions of spirituality goes hand in hand with relieving patient suffering. This is the case because when spiritual concerns evoke the struggle to find meaning in tragedy; for example, the individual seeker potentially feels alone and isolated, and the compassionate presence of the nurse who is available to listen to patient or family concerns holds the potential to transform the isolation of suffering (Younger, 1995). It was around this point that Gwyn acknowledged her one regret about Mr. Warren's care—she turned away from his wife when she needed her presence.

Supporting patient spirituality begins with an exquisitely sensitive perception of the spiritual dimensions of the patient's experience. This does not mean that the nurse must have full understanding about spiritual matters or expertise in the world's religions. However, it does require a receptivity to the spiritual dimension of human experience and the setting aside of the assumption of absolute truth in regard to one's own personal religious beliefs. This is not always easy given the mystery of spiritual matters and the natural tendency to feel fear or threat when faced with the unknown. Further, as evident in Gwyn's story, there are multiple competing demands upon the nurse.

The subtlety of patient spiritual experiences render them easily inhibited, obscured, or overlooked. Reynolds Price described the delicacy of his own spiritual awakenings in his book written for a young man seeking spiritual comfort as he faced the disappointment and agony of his death: "There've been no shows of light, no gleaming illusory messengers, almost no words; and the music that underlies each moment is silent but felt in every cell like a grander pulse beneath my own" (Price, 1999, p. 28). Further, expressions of spirituality are as varied as human experience. For example, patients may encounter as spiritual a line of poetry, a sunset, the birth of a child, a positive medical report, a note from a friend, the touch of a nurse, a call from a grandchild, a verse from a sacred text, a single flower, or the death of another patient.

Gwyn's support for Mr. Warren's spirituality began with her recognition of the importance to Mr. Warren of his family. Knowing that the suddenness and seriousness of his illness was traumatic for the entire family, she explained to them the meaning of the tests he was undergoing. Early in his illness she incorporated the children into his daily care, showing them how to help him walk in the halls and how to assist with his mouth care and shaving. When his kidneys failed and he refused dialysis, it was clear to all that he was dying. In response she did anticipatory teaching so they could know what to expect over the next days.

The day Mr. Warren died, Gwyn was instrumental in creating the circumstances that enabled the family to participate in Mr. Warren's dying experience. First, she gave them guidance. Encouraging them, she said, "Tell him it is OK for him to go. Tell him you will be OK." She stood quietly as each in turn told Mr. Warren good-bye. Second, Gwyn helped create private space for Mr. Warren's dying. Standing guard at the door, she kept staff and visitors out of the room. When the doctor stopped by, she silenced him with a gesture, cueing him into the significance of the moment and enabling his silent and unobtrusive participation in the experience.

As Mr. Warren was dying, Gwyn's support was quiet and, at face value, unremarkable. Noting that "they were all participating in his dying," she left the family alone except for her encouragement to reassure Mr. Warren. She did not try to manage the situation or intrude by taking his vital signs. Recognizing that they were taking their comfort from one another, she did not step into the family circle to offer comfort. Significantly, she simply helped create a space in a noisy and busy hospital for a family-focused, quiet, and—ultimately for her—life-changing experience.

Challenges to Supporting Spirituality

There are multiple challenges to supporting a patient's spirituality. With few exceptions, the settings in which nurses work are defined by medical equipment crowded into small, sterile rooms. In such settings, nurses are pressed for time and must focus on physical concerns (Ross, 1994), making it difficult to notice the subtle spiritual needs of patients.

Personal factors may also threaten the nurse's spiritual care. Some nurses fail to recognize expressions of spirituality or religion that differ from their own (Taylor et al., 1995). These nurses may go so far as to assume that their own spiritual or religious orientation is the only valid approach to spiritual or religious matters. Others fear getting involved in something they do not understand or violating a patient's privacy by mentioning spiritual matters (Laukhuf & Werner, 1998). Some may feel discomfort in matters that are as intimate and private as the spiritual. Still other nurses are confused about their own beliefs and consequently feel they cannot develop skill in spiritual care (Taylor et al., 1995). Nurses may also find that the words commonly associated with spiritual matters such as *love, prayer, agony, meaning, hope, despair,* or *God* are difficult for them to use, especially in settings that are focused on physical, as opposed to spiritual, concerns.

There are also patient challenges to spiritual care. It was easy for Gwyn to recognize and appreciate Mr. Warren's spiritual strengths given his obvious spiritual and religious orientation. Further, his expressions of spirituality were quiet, peaceful, and fully acceptable to Gwyn. However, some patients are not likable and manifest spiritual needs in ways that are loud and demanding. These patients may be totally without family or advocates, save a willing health care provider, and they are filled with pain and anguish. The spiritual suffering of these patients causes anxiety in the nurse who has not acknowledged the darkness in her own life. This anxiety in turn may lead the nurse to disengage from the patient, thereby increasing the patient's isolation and agony. The courage required for spiritual care is great because it entails facing one's own darkness, fears, and agony, thereby positioning the nurse for a careful response to the full range of patient needs.

Given these challenges and the subtle nature of spiritual experiences, responding to patient spirituality is complicated. Movement toward this response involves paying attention. Attention entails engagement in the moment. That is to say, when the nurse focuses attention on a patient, the nurse is engaged with that patient. It is not necessary to understand the variety of patient creeds, doctrines, or forms of spirituality; rather, it is necessary to *notice* the patient's expressions of feelings, questions of meaning, and spiritual affirmations. This requires attention to the patient, receptivity to the patient, and is still further facilitated by a familiarity with one's own spirituality.

Developing spirituality is a life-long process that involves paying attention to your own experiences and asking questions such as, What do I believe about the meaning of life? What do I value in life? or What does it mean to be loving toward another person? (Laukhuf & Werner, 1998). When you begin to ask these questions about your own life, you will have taken the first step toward noticing spirituality in your patient. In turn, as you begin to recognize and honor your patient's spirituality, your own spirituality will grow. In an examination of spiritual care among nurses, Ross (1994) noted that nurses who gave expert spiritual care were aware of the spiritual dimension in their own lives, had experienced personal growth from crises in their own lives, showed a willingness to give of themselves at a deep personal level, and had well-developed skills of sensitivity and perception.

Responses to patient spirituality do not need to be time-consuming or complex. Spiritual care may be as uncomplicated as allowing a family member to stay beyond visiting hours to read a sacred text to a patient or pray with a patient, listening to patients talk about their sense of despair and anguish, involving the clergy or chaplain in patient care, checking frequently on a patient who has just received a life-threatening medical report, gently touching a patient who is fearful of a procedure, or simply not interfering with spiritual rites, as modeled by Gwyn. As with all artful nursing care, the key to spiritual care is to ensure that you respond to the patient's needs, not the needs of the nurse. This is particularly difficult for nurses whose religious beliefs include the assumption of absolute truth in regard to religious or spiritual matters and who hold a desire to share their religious perspective with a suffering patient. Despite these challenges, spiritual care, like physical care, requires a response that is finely tuned to the individual patient's needs and that, like the grief and joy of life, beg for our attention (Tarrant, 1998).

Summary

Awareness of the spiritual aspects of the patient's experience is a vital though subtle and challenging feature of the art of nursing. Spiritual care begins with recognizing the distinctions between spirituality and religion, developing skills in noting the manifestations of spirituality in patients, and knowing that patient's spiritual questions are not problems to be solved by the nurse but opportunities to show compassion and sensitivity. The range of spiritual expression is wide, encompassing feelings of joy, hope, and optimism, as well as sadness and despair. Spiritual care entails paying attention to the patient and experiences in one's own life that evoke spiritual responses.

References

Brussat, F., & Brussat, M.A. (1996). *Spiritual literacy.* New York, NY: Simon & Schuster.

Burkhardt, M.A. (1994). Becoming and connecting: Elements of spirituality for women. *Holistic Nursing Practice 8*(4), 12–21.

Calabria, M.D., & Macrae, J.A. (Eds.). (1994). *Suggestions for thought by Florence Nightingale.* Philadelphia, PA: University of Pennsylvania Press.

Clark, C.C. (1997). Recognizing spiritual needs of orthopaedic patients. *Orthopaedic Nursing, 16*(6), 27–32.

Gaines, E.J. (1993). *A lesson before dying.* New York, NY: Vintage Books.

Gould, S.J. (1999). Dorothy, it's really Oz. *Time,* August 23, p. 59.

Halstead, M.T., & Mickley, R. (1997). Attempting to fathom the unfathomable: Descriptive views of spirituality. *Seminars in Oncology Nursing, 13,* 225–230.

International Code for Nurses. (1973). *Code for nurses, ethical concepts applied to nursing.* Geneva, Switzerland: Author.

Kahn, D.L., & Steeves, R.H. (1994). Spiritual well being: A review of the research literature. *Quality of Life, 2,* 60–64.

Katz, J. (1999). *Running to the mountain.* New York, NY: Villard.

Laukhuf, G., & Werner, H. (1998). Spirituality: The missing link. *Journal of Neuroscience Nursing, 30*(1), 60–67.

Macrae, J. (1995). Nightingale's spiritual philosophy and its significance for modern nursing. *Image, 27,* 8–10.

Mayer, J. (1992). Wholly responsible for a part, or partly responsible for a whole? *Second Opinion, 17*(3), 26–55.

Nolan, P., & Crawford, P. (1997). Towards a rhetoric of spirituality in mental health care. *Journal of Advanced Nursing, 26,* 289–294.

O'Conner, A.P., Wicker, C.A., & Germino, B.B. (1990). Understanding the cancer patient's search for meaning. *Cancer Nursing, 13,* 167–175.

Price, R. (1999). *Letters to a man in the fire.* New York, NY: Scribner.

Ross, L.A. (1994). Spiritual aspects of nursing. *Journal of Advanced Nursing, 19,* 439–447.

Sacks, O. (1984). *A leg to stand on.* New York, NY: Summit Books.

Stiles, M.K. (1994). The shining stranger: Application of the phenomenological method in the investigation of the nurse-family spiritual relationship. *Cancer Nursing, 17,* 18–26.

Sumner, C.H. (1998). Recognizing and responding to spiritual distress. *American Journal of Nursing, 98*(1), 26–30.

Tarrant, J. (1998). *The light inside the dark.* New York, NY: Harper Perennial.

Taylor, E.J., Amenta, M., & Highfield, M. (1995). Spiritual care practices of oncology nurses. *Oncology Nursing Forum, 22,* 31–39.

Verghese, A. (1998). *The tennis partner: A doctor's story of friendship and loss.* New York, NY: HarperCollins.

Walker, A. (1982). *The color purple.* New York, NY: Harcourt Brace Jovanovich.

Watson, J. (1985). *Nursing: human science and human care.* Norwalk, CT: Appleton-Century-Crofts.

Wright, K.B. (1998). Professional, ethical, and legal implications for spiritual care in nursing. *Image, 30,* 81–83.

Younger, J.B. (1995). The alienation of the sufferer. *Advances in Nursing Science, 17*(4), 53–72.

APPLICATION

....

ACTIVITY I
Group Discussion: Analysis of the Story

1. Consider Gwyn's situation when Mrs. Warren approached her with her plea, "What should we do? I cannot imagine how I can survive without him, my life is so closely a part of his. I do not want him to suffer, but I cannot just let him go." Since Gwyn was too busy to talk with Mrs. Warren at this time, what else could she have done to address Mrs. Warren's needs?

2. Mr. Warren never spoke directly about his impending death with Gwyn. Do you think she should have opened this discussion with him? If so, what could she have said. What would you have done?

3. As Mr. Warren was dying, he spoke about going home. What do you think he meant by this? Do you share the religious beliefs reflected in his comments about going home? How would you have reacted to the events that surrounded his dying?

4. What do you think Gwyn meant by the comment, "I continue on what I call a spiritual quest. I have more questions than answers, but I have a new awareness of the spiritual aspect of life"?

5. Discuss your response to the following statement: "As with all artful nursing care, the key to spiritual care is to ensure that you respond to the patient's need, not the needs of the nurse. This is particularly difficult for nurses whose religious beliefs include the assumption of absolute truth in regard to religious or spiritual matters and who hold a desire to share their religious perspective with a suffering patient." What does this mean? When is it appropriate for nurses to share their religious perspective with a patient?

ACTIVITY II
Group Activity: Recognizing Manifestations of Spirituality

1. Working as a group, select one story highlighted in any chapter of this text.

2. Discuss those aspects of the story that are related to patient or nurse spirituality, as the concept has been depicted in this chapter.

ACTIVITY III
Case Analysis with Group Discussion: Responding to Spiritual Needs

You are caring for a patient who has cancer. The patient is 37 years old, is married, and has two children. He is refusing treatment because he does not want to undergo the painful aspects of chemotherapy and radiation. He has been told that he will probably die without treatment. He says, "God will take care of me. If it is my time to die, I will die. If it is not my time to die, He will send a miracle and save me." His wife is frantic and has pleaded with her husband to undergo treatment. She turns to you and says, "Please help me."

GROUP DISCUSSION QUESTIONS

1. Do you share the husband's beliefs about God?

2. What would you say to the wife?

3. How would you feel toward the patient?

4. What would you say to the patient?

5. Would you try to persuade the patient to take treatment, and if so, how would you go about this? Discuss whether it is OK for the nurse to take sides in a situation like this, that is, align with the wife or husband?

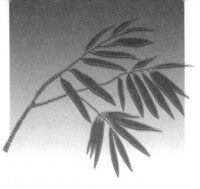

CHAPTER 8

Response of Compassion

Introduction

In a revealing account of her work as an adult nurse practitioner (ANP), Cortney Davis (1997) described how her experience unexpectedly converged with that of a patient. Davis was working in a woman's health clinic when a young, blond, tattooed, 26-week-pregnant drug addict named Ellie walked into the clinic announcing that her water had broken. It was quickly apparent that she had an infection and her baby would die. At the time, Davis silently noted how little she had in common with her patient. Later that day, as she walked to her car after work, she barely escaped an attacker. Shaken, she thought: "I felt as hopeless and as pursued as my patient must have [felt] when I announced that her baby would probably die. [I am] like Ellie . . . no better, no worse" (p. 112).

In a poem about the experience, Davis (1997) wrote:

> I see the woman in the clinic
> turn toward me
> with black eyeliner like thumbprints
> under her eyes, her arms
> opened and scarred by the needle.
> I say, *The baby*
> *will probably not survive.*
> *This is some fucking mess,* she says,
> The man right behind me, my car
> on the far side of the ramp,
> both of us knowing
> that I am a woman like any woman,
> like my patient, like any thin girl
> a scared woman finally squeezes out, just
> skin and hair and this sharp primal smell (pp. 112–113)

Compassion is the core of caring (Wilkes & Wallis, 1998). Indeed, compassion is the touchstone of the art of nursing and is the thread linking the stories in this text. The origin of the word is *co-pati,* meaning to suffer with (Thomasma & Kushner, 1995). Hence, to practice nursing with compassion means to suffer with your patients. As Davis (1997) makes clear in her poem, compassion entails recognizing all aspects of human experience—the light and the dark—in both yourself and the patient. To turn away from the patient is to turn away from yourself. Further, to turn from compassion is to abandon the patient, increase patient loneliness and suffering (Younger, 1995), and reject the heart of the profession of nursing, which is caring for others (Wilkes & Wallis, 1998).

This chapter will examine three aspects of compassion:

- The dance of compassion
- Suffering and compassion
- Empathy and compassion

The Dance of Compassion

Compassion is a complex and challenging dance in which the nurse moves "back and forth with the patient on cue in a caring receptivity" (Younger, 1995, p. 69). The dance begins with the recognition of suffering and requires overcoming a natural inclination to turn away from suffering, particularly when the patient is unattractive or even repulsive. Compassion helps the nurse to rise above the revulsion evoked by foul-smelling dressings, putrid wounds, necrotic tissue, and the distinct smell of death, and gently and tenderly care for another (Kushner, 1995). Such a nurse "can draw the pus out of a carbuncle and with his gaze alone, turn it into a jewel" (Selzer, 1993, p. 56).

Physician Richard Selzer, whose 21-day coma made him totally dependent on the skills and compassion of nurses and physicians, observed in an interview following his recovery that without compassion for persons with failing bodies, "We have no way of taking care of each other. A caregiver . . . needs to have the wisdom to see beyond the wounds of the flesh" (Kushner, 1995, p. 496). Recalling his failing body as "something that even I would not want to touch," Selzer observed, "Not so the nurses—Maureen, Linda, Heather. Beautifully serene, they continue to stroke and massage [me], to wipe away all stains, to bathe and dress [me] in clean linen" (Selzer, 1994, p. 35). In short, Selzer's nurses saw beyond his failing body to his essence as a suffering individual.

While the *recognition* of suffering is the first step in the dance of compassion, the second step involves a decision *not* to turn away but to enter *into* the suffering with the patient (Younger, 1995). This means that the nurse feels what the other feels—vulnerability, loss, alienation, terror. And thus the nurse understands what the patient values and needs (Dougherty & Purtilo, 1995). Recall in Chapter 5 Jana's efforts on behalf of Margaret who wanted TPN to sustain her life until the reconciliation with her daughter was complete. Jana did not simply *understand* that Margaret wanted TPN; she *felt* her longing for reconciliation with her daughter. She entered into and became a part of Margaret's experience.

The third step in the dance of compassion involves the desire to do something about the patient's suffering. The compassionate nurse seeks to alleviate suffering or to support the person by living through the experience with him (Dougherty & Purtilo, 1995). Jana translated her compassion into action: she was willing to help and to go out of her way to relieve Margaret's suffering (Thomasma & Kusher, 1995). Further, she sustained those actions through weeks of intensive physical care.

Compassionate involvement by the nurse may be exhibited in various responses including advocacy, illustrated by Jana's story; or a quiet, faithful, and attuned nurse presence, illustrated by Elizabeth's care of her dying patient Leah in Chapter 4; or by the quiet presence of the nurse, as Edith illustrates in Chapter 9. Compassionate actions range from simple things like calling the doctor to get pain medication, making a phone call for a patient, or getting a cup of coffee for a family member, to stopping by the local animal shelter to see if the missing cat belonging to your worried homebound elderly patient is there. Whatever the activity, the link to compassion lies in the nurse's recognition that she is connected to the patient by shared human experience (Younger, 1995).

Compassion is always without judgment, for judging a patient separates him from the nurse. Just as she does not recoil from draining wounds, the compassionate nurse does not recoil from or judge angry, depressed, or horrified patients. Acceptance comes from the recognition that the nurse, like her patient, is capable of producing foul-smelling drainage and feeling anger, rage, and horror.

Compassion cannot be extended to a patient whom the nurse finds unattractive unless the nurse has accepted within herself the very possibilities that she finds repugnant or frightening in the patient. In other words, compassion depends upon the ability to recognize and accept both the light *and* the dark in experience. The dark feelings and tragedies that befall the patient could also fall upon the nurse (Younger, 1995). Further, the dark actions and feelings that arise *from* patients could also arise from the nurse. Acknowledgment of the light and the dark in our lives ties us to all of ourselves and makes possible compassion for all patients, regardless of their physical or emotional conditions. Younger (1995) described this process when she wrote, "In a compassionate embrace of the dark side of reality, we become bearers of the light. We open to the other—the strange, the weak, the sinful, the despised—and simply through including the dark, we transmute it" (1995, p. 65).

Elizabeth (in Chapter 4) illustrated this when, in caring for her dying patient Leah, she recognized that she herself was not immune to such tragedy. Elizabeth did not deny the reality that mothers sometimes die and leave a small child. Because Elizabeth acknowledged the darkness in human experience, she did not have to pretend that Leah's horror was unreal or dismiss it with simplistic reassurance. Elizabeth could suffer with Leah at the point of Leah's greatest pain and conclude, "I do believe my presence helped her. Presence can help when the pain is very deep. Presence can make things a little better."

Suffering and Compassion

Suffering may be thought of as "the distress brought about by the actual or perceived impending threat to the integrity or continued existence of the whole person" (Cassell, 1991, p. 24). The whole person involves more than the physical existence; it also involves a sense that one is spiritually and emotionally intact. Thus physical pain that does not threaten the integrity of the patient—for example, the pain of childbirth—does not cause suffering. However, events that put life at risk like a diagnosis of cancer or the news that one is HIV positive evoke suffering. Likewise, events that threaten one's continuity or way of life, like the loss of a job, the birth of a handicapped child, or the death of a loved one, evoke suffering. The realization that these life-altering events are not under one's control contributes to the suffering (Younger, 1995).

Suffering separates the sufferer from others. In part that is because the experience of suffering is vastly different for the sufferer and the one who observes the sufferer. For the suffering patient, physical or spiritual pain cannot be avoided, wished away, or denied. Yet the observing nurse may ignore or deny the existence of the pain. For the sufferer, pain is certain, immediate, and threatening; for the observer, the very existence of the pain may be doubted (Scarry, 1985). In her classic book about pain Scarry writes, "Thus pain comes *unsharably* [italics added] into our midst as at once that which cannot be denied and that which cannot be confirmed" (p. 4). Hence, the first challenge to the nurse faced with patient suffering is to close the gap created by the unsharable nature of suffering.

Compassion is further challenged by the unspeakable nature of suffering (Younger, 1995). There is no language to describe the experience of suffering

(Scarry, 1985). Inarticulate, the sufferer often expresses his suffering through silent withdrawal, moans, groans, or tortured cries. When there are no words to describe suffering, the compassionate nurse enters into the patient's suffering by a respectful silence (Dougherty & Purtilo, 1995) or by acknowledging it with words like "I am here" or "I will be with you in this experience." Such efforts to reach out show the patient that the nurse is available to enter into the experience with the patient.

By acknowledging the patient's suffering, the nurse shifts the private and isolating experience of suffering into a shared experience. The patient may then be able to find words to speak the unspeakable, moving out of her own isolation. Younger (1995) says, "If people cannot speak about their affliction, they will be destroyed by it or swallowed up by apathy. It is not important where they find the language or what form it takes, but it is very important that the language be found" (p. 70).

In Chapter 5 Jana helped the patient give voice to suffering when faced with death. Her patient Margaret was initially silent. Jana remained engaged with her and invited her responses. Eventually Margaret spoke of her fears about her illness, said what she needed, and with Jana's help explored ways to meet her needs. However, Margaret's needs could not be met until she could articulate her suffering over her impending death and estrangement from her daughter. Working with Jana, she could then identify a way to alleviate her suffering. Her determination to live until she became reconciled with her daughter brought new meaning to her suffering.

Empathy and Compassion

Rawnsley's (1990) account of a mother's response to her dying daughter illustrates how empathy enables compassion. Angela, the daughter, was close to death. She opened her eyes and asked,

> "'Momma, are you here?' Her mother took her hand. 'Yes, I am here,' she answered. A few minutes later Angela asked, 'Momma, am I dead yet?' Her mother moved to the bed and stroked her daughter's arm. 'Angela,' she said, 'you are here with me.' Angela stirred again, 'Are we dead together, Momma?' There was a brief hesitation, then her mother spoke softly, 'Yes, Angela, we are together.'" (p. 44)

Empathy gives rise to the response of compassion. Empathy occurs when the nurse views the patient's experience from the patient's perspective and conveys his understanding without judgment. This requires setting aside perceptions of "how this experience would be for me" (Wiseman, 1996). Carl Rogers (1957) described empathy as the ability to sense the world of the patient as if it were one's own while holding onto the "as if" quality of the experience. In Rawnsley's story, the mother recognized her daughter's need for her presence and offered solace in her affirmation, "We are together." The mother understood her child's fear and responded accordingly, without losing sight of the fact that the dying experience was her daughter's, not her own. Had she missed the "as if" quality of empathy, she would have been unable to respond to her daughter's need because of her own pain.

It is natural for a mother to feel empathy for a daughter, since empathy easily arises from feelings of love and mutuality built upon shared experiences. Likewise, empathy is easy for a nurse who shares experiences with a patient because of similarities in gender, social class, or race (Olsen, 1991). Think about your own practice and how easy it is to feel a kinship with patients who are like you or who remind you of someone you love. Empathy arising from mutually shared experiences, however, extends to a relatively narrow range of patients.

Empathy can also arise from recognition of shared feelings (Olsen, 1991). For example, the nurse may recognize how a grieving wife feels because the nurse has had similar feelings in response to his own losses. This form of empathy is also relatively easily evoked in a sensitive, caring nurse.

The greatest challenge is to feel empathy when there is no readily apparent mutuality with a patient. The nurse does not feel an easy kinship with all patients. Imagine the challenge of empathizing with a patient who is a rapist or murderer, or even with a patient who is rude to everyone. With such patients, empathy comes from a recognition that regardless of gender, ethnicity, temperament, or behavior, nurses have in common with all patients the "mutuality that arises from a shared humanness" (Olsen, 1991, p. 70). In other words, nurses and patients have in common the experience of being human and because of this commonality they share human frailties and vulnerabilities. Recognition of our shared human experience provides the means for empathy and makes a compassionate response available to all patients, including patients whose cultural background, education, experiences, beliefs, and values differ from those of the nurse (Price & Archbold, 1997).

The story below illustrates compassion for a patient with whom, at first glance, the nurse had little in common. Mark recognized unspoken suffering, saw the patient as an individual who was unique and who shared similarities with him, and entered into the patient's experience to respond with compassion.

Mark's Story

Rick grew up in a southern university town, the son of a physician father and a mother who was a university professor. His childhood was happy and included church attendance with his family, vacations, summer camps, and activities with his brother and their friends.

Rick was a bright student. In high school he took top honors in all the math contests in his school and in the local community. During his senior year, however, Rick's grades began to decline and he lost interest in his friends. He would spend hours in his room listening to music and smoking cigarettes. Efforts by his parents to talk to him were met with hostility and rejection. Worried, his parents finally persuaded Rick to go with them to see a therapist who, after several family sessions, concluded that Rick was suffering from a difficult adolescence that he would outgrow.

When Rick left the support and familiarity of home to go to college, his appearance became unkempt and disheveled, and his behavior became bizarre. He would walk up to strangers on campus and ask if they were extraterrestrials or if they knew the ultimate mathematical solution to the problems of the universe. One evening he went out on the balcony of the eighth floor of his dorm and climbed on the railing so he could be "closer to God." His roommate called the campus police, who took Rick to the emergency room of the local hospital, where he was admitted for psychiatric evaluation.

After several days in the hospital, it was apparent that Rick was having auditory hallucinations. He heard voices saying that he had been chosen by God to save the universe through mathematical formulas. It was important, Rick reported, to stay in touch with the voice of God through his mathematical skills.

Diagnosed with undifferentiated schizophrenia, Rick responded well to medication and within ten days was discharged from the hospital to his parents' home. Unable to tolerate the stress of school, he withdrew. Over the next five years he had frequent hospital admissions, necessitated in large part by failure to take his medicine consistently. Each time Rick relapsed it became harder to get his symptoms under control.

Eventually Rick's insurance ran out, and he was admitted to the state hospital, where Mark became his nurse. "Rick was 24 when I met him," Mark recalled. "Because he was acutely psychotic, he had been sent to a locked ward on the rehabilitation unit where I worked. A thin, poorly groomed young man, he was gesturing and responding aloud to hallucinations. His agitation was profound, evident in his pacing and the intensity of his responses to the hallucinations. Periodically, he would suddenly stand still and with a look of confusion put his hands over his face, and shout, 'No! No! That's not the way.' He would not let anyone come physically close to him without striking out. During this phase of his illness, we medicated him heavily but even then he could not get much relief. He paced much of the night. I was drawn to Rick by the tragedy of his illness—he had been a bright, attractive, and happy young man only a few years earlier, anticipating a normal life. Now his dreams were shattered continually by this terrible illness. He could never expect to be free from the threat of relapse. I could have had this disease, or someone I loved. Because of my appreciation of his suffering, I needed to help him."

The treatment plan focused on stabilizing Rick with medications and then helping him learn to continue taking his medications after discharge. Mark explained, "The new drugs are quite effective and easier to tolerate than the older drugs. However, as patients begin to feel better on the medications, they often stop taking them. Helping patients gain insight into the need for continued medication therapy after discharge takes time."

Mark saw Rick each day, monitoring his response to his medications, assessing for side effects, and evaluating the content and severity of his hallucinations and delusions. Mark mostly observed Rick, asked a few questions, and, when Rick could tolerate it, helped with Rick's bathing and grooming. Preoccupied with his symptoms, Rick rarely spoke. Mark explained, "When patients are acutely psychotic, they cannot tolerate much interaction. However, it is important to show up each day and acknowledge the patient. He needed to be sure I was there for him, and I needed to be there to see how he was coping. I did not need any response from him except to see a remission in his acute agitation, which did occur over several days."

As Rick improved, Mark would occasionally take him off the locked ward for a walk. Once they were strolling on the grounds and a light breeze moved through the trees. Noting this, the usually quiet Rick remarked, "I haven't noticed the leaves on the trees in years. Look at them move. They are beautiful." Mark recalled, "I suddenly realized that something as available to me as the beauty of nature had been lost to Rick and now, for the moment, recovered. His comment touched me and gave me a better understanding of his extreme isolation. Even though he was not often communicative, I realized that he was touched by the same event that moved me—the subtlety of the wind in the leaves. I felt that our worlds had moved a little closer: we shared an appreciation for the beauty in nature."

Within two weeks Rick's thought processes cleared enough to transfer him to an open ward on the rehabilitation unit; he was free now to move about the hospital and grounds. Gradually Rick began to talk a little with Mark, although he remained guarded. In response, Mark made himself more available to his patient. "I knew he was beginning to think more clearly and might tell me more about himself," Mark recalled.

While Rick rarely talked directly about his feelings, indirectly he revealed his shame about his illness. He spoke of his brother who was healthy, married, and had children, remarking that he was not welcome in his brother's home because his brother and his wife were afraid he would hurt the children. He noted his parents' reluctance to take him out in public to shop or to a restaurant.

Mark recognized in these remarks Rick's sense that he was less deserving than his brother and needed acceptance by his parents. "When he was delusional—which was often—he would ask me if he were married or whether he was engaged," said Mark. "Like all of us, he longed for a normal life. Unlike many of us, however, he had to begin by overcoming stigma, even with his family. I cranked up my efforts to validate him in any way that I could."

As Rick improved he began to mingle a bit with other patients, although he rarely initiated contact with anyone. Once Mark observed Rick break this pattern of self-isolation when an elderly patient was trying to purchase a soda from the drink machine. Recognizing that the man needed help, Rick approached him. The man did not have enough money for a drink, so Rick and the elderly patient pooled their resources and bought a soda, which they then shared. Mark said, "This generous response was so touching. Rick had so little, yet he reached out to someone else. This gave me a new glimpse into my patient, whose desires to be of service to others and to be needed were similar to my own. Despite the challenges of his illness, he was kind and generous. I wanted to help him recognize these attributes within the constraints of his illness."

Rick's reticence was less obvious when student nurses came to the unit for clinical experiences. Occasionally Rick would initiate contact with the students and, attracted to one of the young women, would flirt with her. "It was touching to notice his attraction and sad to recognize how unlikely he was to ever have a normal relationship with a woman," said Mark. "I continued to try to talk with him. I knew that as he got better, he would increasingly recognize his isolation. I wanted him to feel that he was not alone."

After several contacts with the student nurses, Rick began to believe that he himself was a nurse. Mark said, "It was hard to challenge his delusion without diminishing his fragile sense of self-worth. When he could tolerate it, I would try to drive a little doubt into the delusion. It was tricky because the delusion provided a sense of worth, which he needed me to reinforce."

To bolster his belief that he was a nurse, Rick wrote to the state Board of Nursing. The official reply came, stating that there was no record indicating Rick was a nurse. Rick brought this letter to Mark, questioning its meaning. Mark reinforced the contents of the letter: "You are not a nurse. However, you are like a nurse in many ways. You are smart, you are kind, and you want to help others. I have seen your kindness."

Rick sat passively as Mark talked. Then he became agitated and declared, "I'm leaving this place. I'll never get well. I'm walking. I'm heading to the next town if I need to, but I'm leaving this place. You can't keep me here." Startled, Mark realized that his efforts to help Rick see reality had led to anger and frustration.

"Let's think about this together, Rick," Mark replied. "I understand how badly you want to be a nurse. I know this letter is a disappointment to you, but recognizing that you are not a nurse is an important part of getting better."

Not answering, Rick continued his pacing. Mark went on, "I know you want to get out of the hospital. Walking, however, will not get you closer to your goal of being discharged. What do you think will happen when you start walking down the highway to the next town?"

"Nothing," Rick responded.

"What happened last week when Sadie [another patient] left the grounds? How far did she get?" Mark asked.

"Not too far, but I'm faster and smarter than Sadie," Rick said.

"This is true," Mark said. "However, if you walk and the police pick you up, like Sadie you will have to go to the locked ward. Let's think of other ways to reach your goal of discharge. I can help you," Mark concluded.

"I can't think of much," a despondent Rick realized.

Mark recalled, "I saw a bright young man whose dreams were constantly destroyed by illness. I recalled my own disappointments and saw myself in him; I wanted to comfort him. So I just told him what was in my heart. I looked at Rick and I said, 'Rick, you are a brave young man. I have great respect for you.'"

Hearing Mark's encouragement, Rick's hand went to his quivering mouth and his eyes filled with tears. He excused himself and retreated to the bathroom to compose himself.

"That was a real breakthrough for Rick," Mark observed. "This rare show of emotion told me that Rick heard my words, was touched by them, and recognized my respect for him. I hoped that at that point he began to see his own decency and value. I was touched when he allowed me to share this brief human connection with him."

The next letter Rick wrote was to the local community college, requesting a catalogue of courses. Mark brought Rick several math texts, donated by the local used book store, and despite his limited ability to concentrate, Rick began to spend a few minutes each day working math problems. He took great delight in posing problems for the nursing students, who often could not solve the mathematical puzzles he put forward.

As Rick approached discharge, he was stable but not symptom free. He still heard voices and had delusions. However, he was learning to recognize the voices as a part of his illness, and he was getting better at ignoring them. He was also becoming skilled at questioning his delusions.

After nine weeks on the rehabilitation unit, Rick was discharged to a community-supported group home where he had his own room, assistance with meals, and reminders to take his medications. He quickly mastered the public transportation system and joined the community clubhouse for persons with severe and persistent mental illness (SPMI). With help from the clubhouse staff, Rick enrolled in a math course and earned a grade of B.

Over the next three years, Rick relapsed three times while on his medications and required brief hospitalizations to readjust the medications. During each hospitalization, Mark was Rick's primary nurse. "He began to trust me except when he was acutely psychotic and could trust no one," Mark said.

Outside the hospital, Rick stayed in touch with Mark through occasional phone calls and letters. Continuing to adjust to his illness, Rick took more math courses and participated in the clubhouse activities. Eventually he moved to his own apartment in a community-supported complex where several of his companions from the clubhouse also lived. Together these men frequented the local coffeehouses and got together to watch videos and listen to music. Eventually Rick also managed to work for several hours each day with a supervised ground crew at the local college, in a work program sponsored by the clubhouse. During this time, whenever he contacted Mark, he would say he still heard voices but was learning to live with them. "I don't know how he did it," Mark noted. "I would have given up long ago. His life was constricted and hard, but he managed to find enough meaning to take occasional courses and do limited work. Each time I had contact with him, I was touched by his ability to keep on keeping on."

Mark recalled, "Several months after Rick's last hospitalization, I was walking downtown with my young daughter and we ran into Rick, who greeted me in a loud, booming voice. I introduced him to my daughter, and we walked together for a few blocks. As we approached the ice cream shop, I announced that it was my destination, to which Rick responded, 'Well, I'm sorry I can't join you, but I have to go to work.' I was pleased that Rick had a job and things to do, and I was moved once again by his courage. More importantly, I was happy to note that he assumed he would be welcome to join my daughter and me in an ice cream. Perhaps he was finally beginning to appreciate what he had to offer."

Enacting Artful Nursing

Mark's story demonstrates the dance of compassion. Mark recognized Rick's suffering, Mark got to know Rick as an individual, and Mark took action on Rick's behalf to relieve his suffering. Three features of compassion highlighted in Mark's story are
- Recognizing suffering
- Seeing patient individuality
- Alleviating suffering

RECOGNIZING SUFFERING

Schizophrenia brings extreme suffering to patients and families. The disease disrupts one's understanding of oneself and isolates one from others. Few patients manage to avoid chronic symptoms that wax and wane, frustration with medications that reduce symptoms but often bring troubling side effects, or the stigma that cuts the patient off from full acceptance in society. For patients with schizophrenia there are days when there is no comfort. For many, voices and delusions continue, defying the best efforts of psychiatrists working with new drugs. Doors are closed to these patients and access to normal activities lost as they struggle with a disease that isolates them; they experience lonely weekends and long, empty holidays (Riley, 1997). Adding to their suffering is the fact that the suffering often goes unrecognized by lay persons and professionals, whose failures of compassion sometimes have devastating outcomes (Kiefer, 1997; Sharav & Sharav, 1997).

The first step in compassion begins with recognizing the suffering of the patient. In Mark's story, obstacles to compassion such as the natural tendency to turn away from what is unattractive, the difficulty that all patients have in giving voice to suffering, and the nonsufferer's doubts of the claims of the sufferer were compounded by the nature of Rick's illness. To appreciate Rick's suffering, Mark had to become engaged with a patient whose disordered thought processes, agitated behavior, and unkempt appearance created vast distance between them. Despite this distance, Mark's awareness of how deeply patients with uncontrolled schizophrenia suffer drew him to Rick.

Mark's understanding of what separated *and* connected the two men was key. Mark knew that Rick's disordered thinking, his pacing and anxiety, his look of confusion when he stopped his pacing and listened to the voices, and his poor grooming created barriers between Rick and others. Mark did not require that Rick look and behave like him nor share his values. Rather, Mark imagined how it would be to have schizophrenia. Seeing his unkempt, thin, agitated patient pacing and gesticulating in response to his hallucinations, Mark was drawn to Rick by his recognition of pain, and he wanted to help.

To help Rick, Mark had to see beyond the obvious. When Rick observed the leaves moving in the wind, Mark saw someone who, like himself, responded to the beauty of nature. He also saw a young man for whom this source of comfort had long been unavailable, and he recognized this absence as pain. On hearing Rick's delusional thoughts, Mark looked for their meaning and the clues they provided to Rick's needs. Rather than seeing Rick as simply delusional and confused, Mark "saw a bright young man whose dreams were destroyed by illness."

SEEING PATIENT INDIVIDUALITY

Mark's capacity to see Rick's individuality was key to the recognition of Rick's suffering. Resisting the temptation to place Rick in the anonymous and broad category of severely and persistently mentally ill persons, Mark sought to understand Rick's world. Rick could not speak directly of his pain, so Mark silently watched and listened for clues about his patient. Observing Rick's behavior and his delusions and hallucinations, Mark caught a glimpse of Rick's longings, needs, and values. He recognized Rick's need for comfort in his pacing and agitation. As Rick spoke about his parents' reluctance to take him out in public, Mark recognized his need for acceptance. Rick's longing for a normal life was evident in his references to his healthy brother and the fact that he was not welcome in his brother's home. His readiness to help the older man purchase a soda showed Rick's generous nature and his wish to be helpful. His flirtations with the student nurses and his delusions about being engaged or married revealed his longing to be loved.

Mark's thoughtful observation of his patient was more than a skilled assessment. He desired to *understand* Rick's suffering. As Mark came to know Rick, his knowledge shed light on the meaning to Rick of his illness and the accompanying pain, guiding Mark's responses to Rick. For example, knowing Rick's intelligence and his longing to be accepted by the student nurses helped Mark understand Rick's despair when he received the letter from the Board of Nursing stating that he was not a nurse. This knowledge also led Mark to bring in the math books for Rick and to encourage Rick to enjoy his skills in math.

Finally, Mark was able to recognize himself in Rick. When the two noticed the leaves moving in the wind, Mark observed, "I moved a bit closer to understanding his world." When Rick's frustration and disappointment surfaced in the face of his rejection from the Board of Nursing, Mark's recollection of his own disappointments moved him to comfort his patient.

ALLEVIATING SUFFERING

Taking action to alleviate suffering depends upon the recognition of suffering and is guided by knowledge of the patient. Mark tried to relieve Rick's suffering and isolation based on cues from Rick. Early in their relationship, when Rick was preoccupied with his hallucinations and acutely psychotic, Mark was faithful in his presence. He showed up. Rick's tolerance for interactions was limited, so Mark quietly went about assessing Rick's symptoms and response to his medications, demanding and expecting little from his acutely ill patient. "Showing up and acknowledging the patient is important," Mark noted.

As Rick's symptoms and agitation began to subside, the evidence of his suffering diminished but the source of his suffering—his disease—remained. Rather than backing away as his patient's agitation subsided, Mark stepped up his interactions with his patient, noting that as Rick got better, he was more likely to "recognize his differences, increasing his sense of isolation from others."

Rick's "suffering work"—which Emerson (1986) has described as the work that moves the patient through a painful situation to a place of healing—took a dramatic leap forward when he took the letter from the Board of Nursing to Mark. Taking his lead from his patient, Mark confronted Rick: "You are not a nurse," he said. Aware that Rick's delusion was providing a sense of worth, Mark then pointed out the ways in which Rick was similar to nurses: he was smart, kind, and caring. His delusion fractured, Rick's anger and frustration escalated and he announced that he was leaving the hospital. Recognizing the loss Rick faced in giving up his delusion, Mark spoke from his heart, "You are a brave young man. I have great respect for you." Instead, Mark could have threatened: "If you leave the grounds, we will lock you up," effectively silencing and further isolating his patient.

Challenges to Compassion

Compassion is at the heart of nursing: this is evident in the stories in this text. However, the requirements of compassion are imposing and include a willingness to enter into pain-filled experiences with patients who are themselves sometimes unattractive. Further, compassion requires the recognition of one's involvement with all of humankind and knowledge of the "nature of life itself and its vicissitudes" (Younger, 1995, p. 71). In short, compassion is a finely developed human response with impressive challenges.

Heavy workloads and limited time may affect the nurse's willingness to extend compassion to patients. Further, a phenomenon called compassion fatigue, or the emotional burden that results when one is overexposed to patient tragedies (Schwam, 1998), may make the nurse reluctant to extend compassion.

Certainly the emotional burden of compassion becomes heavy at times, and compassionate nurses require exquisite ability to care for the self. (Chapter 10 of this text offers a discussion of the art of caring for oneself.) The ability to distinguish between the patient's experience and your own is central. Because this ability can only be acquired through experience, there will be times when you will find yourself overinvolved or uninvolved. Both extremes lead to further suffering for the patient and dissatisfaction for the nurse.

Compassion always requires some emotional investment, along with a recognition that in fundamental human ways the patient does not differ from the nurse (Younger, 1995). Some nurses are constrained in their compassion by their own discomfort with opening themselves to a patient's suffering. A compassionate response is difficult for many individuals, and some nurses are inevitably less compassionate than others.

There are also patients who resist expressions of compassion and who may be withdrawn or hostile, or arrogantly reject the nurse. Patients have the prerogative to refuse compassion offered by the nurse and to remain isolated in their suffering. Nevertheless, given the commitment of nurses to relieve suffering, compassion is a moral duty of every nurse (Dougherty & Purtilo, 1995).

There are also patients who seem undeserving of compassion. In a movie entitled *Dead Man Walking*, a nun offers her compassionate presence to a convicted murderer awaiting his execution. The murderer does not "deserve" the nun's compassion. However, as the movie unfolds, these two unlikely characters become bound by their shared acknowledgment of the tragedies of life. Their relationship is, in an emotional sense, life-saving for the condemned man.

Despite the moral requirements of compassion and your best intentions, there will be some patients for whom you find compassion difficult. There will also be times when you are not able to feel compassion because of your own unmet needs. While you will not feel compassion for every patient you encounter, it is essential to provide competent care to all patients and to avoid behaviors or attitudes that increase patient suffering. If this is impossible with a patient, you should find another nurse to care for that patient and take responsibility for getting your own needs met.

Among nursing students, a major constraint to developing compassion is school requirements. Students can feel so overwhelmed by school pressures and fear of failure that they "forget" the ways in which all humans, including students, teachers, and patients, are connected. Further, if students do not have the benefit of a compassionate teacher, compassion may fall aside. There is no simple antidote to the challenges to compassion imposed by the stress of nursing school, just as there is no easy answer to the other challenges to compassion. However, aligning oneself with a compassionate colleague is one way to remember the essential ingredient of compassion: at a basic human level, the nurse does not differ from the patient and the student does not differ from the teacher.

Summary

Compassion is at the heart of artful nursing. The dance of compassion involves the recognition of patient suffering, the choice to enter into the patient's experience, and the desire to act to relieve the patient's suffering. Actions can take multiple forms, ranging from advocacy to simply being with a patient. Compassion can arise from the acknowledgment of shared experiences or emotions, or at the highest level, the "mutuality that arises from a shared humanness" (Olsen, 1991, p. 70). Compassion requires courage and commitment, and offers the nurse the satisfaction of sharing deeply felt human experiences.

References

Cassell, E.J. (1991). Recognizing suffering. *Hastings Center Report, May–June,* 24–31.

Davis, C. (1997). Poetry about patients: Hearing the nurse's voice. *Journal of Medical Humanities, 18,* 111–125.

Dougherty, C.J., & Purtilo, R. (1995). Physicians' duty of compassion. *Cambridge Quarterly of Healthcare Ethics, 4,* 426–433.

Emerson, J.G. (1986). *Suffering: Its meaning and ministry.* Nashville, Tenn.: Abingdon Press.

Kiefer, F. (1997). Seclusion and restraints. *The Journal of the California Alliance for the Mentally Ill, 8,* 31–36.

Kushner, T. (1995). CQ Interview: Richard Selzer on death, resurrection, and compassion. *Cambridge Quarterly of Healthcare Ethics, 4,* 494–498.

Olsen, D.P. (1991). Empathy as an ethical and philosophical basis for nursing. *Advances in Nursing Science, 1,* 62–75.

Price, V., & Archbold, J. (1997). What's it all about, empathy? *Nurse Education Today, 17,* 106–110.

Rawnsley, M. (1990). Of human bonding: The context of nursing as caring. *Advances in Nursing Science, 13,* 41–48.

Riley, B.J. (1997). Bart. *The Journal of the California Alliance for the Mentally Ill, 8,* 69–72.

Rogers, C. (1957). The necessary and sufficient conditions of therapeutic change. *Journal of Consulting Psychology, 21,* 95–103.

Scarry, E. (1985). *The body in pain.* New York: Oxford University Press.

Schwam, K. (1998). The phenomenon of compassion fatigue in perioperative nursing. *AORN Journal, 68*(4), 642–648.

Selzer, R. (1994). *Raising the dead.* New York: Whittle Books in association with Viking Press.

Sharav, B., & Sharav, I. (1997). Ami, our son, died because of mismanaged care. *The Journal of the California Alliance for the Mentally Ill, 8,* 37–41.

Thomasma, D.C., & Kushner, T. (1995). A dialogue on compassion and supererogation in medicine. *Cambridge Quarterly of Healthcare Ethics, 4,* 415–425.

Wilkes, L.M., & Wallis, M.C. (1998). A model of professional nurse caring: Nursing students' experience. *Journal of Advanced Nursing, 27,* 582–589.

Wiseman, T. (1996). A concept analysis of empathy. *Journal of Advanced Nursing, 23,* 1162–1167.

Younger, J.B. (1995). The alienation of the sufferer. *Advances in Nursing Science, 17,* 53–72.

APPLICATION

....

ACTIVITY I
Group Discussion: Analysis of the Story

1. Discuss the ways in which Mark's compassion for Rick influenced his assessment of his patient. In other words, which aspects of Rick's experience were highlighted by Mark's compassionate view of his patient?

2. What would you have done when Rick told Mark that he was going to run away from the hospital? What would a typical nursing response be to this revelation by a patient? Discuss how Mark's response differed from the typical nursing response to this threat by a patient and the role of compassion in Mark's response.

3. What do you think enabled Mark to feel compassion for Rick and to see beyond Rick's psychotic behavior and unkempt appearance to recognize his basic human needs?

ACTIVITY II
Case Analysis with Group Discussion and Self-Reflection: Exploring Obstacles to Compassion

You are a student nurse working with a preceptor who is a home health nurse. Together you visit a young man who has HIV disease and who is receiving follow-up care after emergency surgery for a bowel obstruction. The patient does not have AIDS. As you prepare to leave, the patient asks your preceptor, "When can I resume sex?" The nurse explains the usual postoperative recovery trajectory and then asks, "What kind of protection do you use when you have sex?"

"I use condoms," the patient replies. Sheepishly, he continues, "For a long time I didn't use anything, even though I knew I was HIV positive. I just didn't tell my partners because I figured they wouldn't have sex with me if they knew, and I needed the intimacy of sexual experiences. But now I use a condom because I figured I might catch another sexually transmitted disease (STD) if I didn't."

The preceptor reinforces the patient's current practice of using a condom during sex and then the two of you leave. As you drive to the next patient's home, you ask the preceptor, "How do you take care of someone like that who is so selfish? I can't believe he didn't tell his partners he was HIV positive and didn't use protection. I wonder how many people he infected."

GROUP DISCUSSION QUESTIONS

Compassion is an ideal toward which the expert nurse strives. However, all nurses lack compassion at times.

1. List some reasons why nurses may not demonstrate compassion.

2. What is it about yourself that may prevent you from being compassionate?

3. What is it about the work setting that may prevent you from being compassionate?

4. Discuss ways to overcome patient, nurse, or setting obstacles to compassion.

SELF-REFLECTION QUESTIONS

1. What would you have said to this patient in response to his revelation that he had unprotected sex knowing he had HIV disease?

2. List any positive traits you see in this young man.

3. Which of these traits are similar to traits in you?

4. How do you express these traits in your life?

5. List the traits in this young man that you see as negative.

6. Which of these negative traits are similar to traits in your life?

7. How do you express these traits in your life?

8. How would you describe the fears that might have influenced this patient's decision not to use a condom?

9. Identify feelings or traits that you have in common with this patient that could serve as a basis for your compassion for him.

ACTIVITY III
Group Discussion: Exploring Compassion

1. Discuss the characteristics of patients for whom you think it will be easy for you to feel compassion.

2. What is it about these patients that makes it easy to feel compassion?

3. Discuss the characteristics of patients for whom you think it will be difficult for you to feel compassion.

4. What is it about these patients that makes it difficult to feel compassion?

ACTIVITY IV
Group Discussion: Suffering and Compassion

The following questions are designed to stimulate your thinking about compassion.

1. Discuss how compassion for patients affects the nurse.

2. Why do you think good people must suffer?

3. What does it mean to find meaning in suffering?

4. How does someone find meaning in suffering?

5. How does watching a movie, like *Dead Man Walking*, or reading short stories, novels, or poetry, enhance your understanding of suffering and compassion?

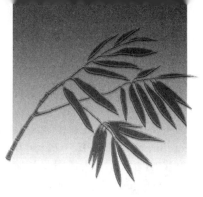

CHAPTER 9

The Presence
of the Nurse

Introduction

The patient lay perfectly still. He was a thin, handsome, young man with long, curling eyelashes. He had just been admitted to the surgical intensive care unit (SICU) following a double lung transplant. Unlike most patients immediately after surgery, he was awake and occasionally alert. The patient had four chest tubes, multiple dressings, nasogastric and endotracheal tubes, and a urinary catheter. The nurse at the bedside was busy checking his drains, measuring the output, monitoring lab values, taking notes, and attending to his numerous peripheral and central lines. Attentive to the patient, she was oblivious to the residents, nurses, and social worker who stopped by to check on a man they had come to know while he waited for his new lungs.

As the nurse worked, she would touch his head or hands, rubbing them and crooning, "You're doing fine." When the patient resisted, shaking his head "No," the nurse responded, "Oh, you're hurting. I'll give you some morphine." Relieved, the patient closed his eyes. Working with his lines and drains, she noted that he had slipped his foot from his covers. "You're too hot?" she asked. He nodded, "Yes," and she removed a blanket, soothing his forehead as she straightened his covers. He roused briefly and she said, "Your brother and parents are here; can they come in to see you?" "Yes," he nodded, and she signaled to the family to enter.

His mother came into the room sobbing. The nurse turned to her and said, "Tell me." In an uncertain voice, his mother said, "I am so hopeful and so afraid." "Yes, I know. I understand," the nurse said as she touched her arm and directed the mother, "Hold his hand, it's OK to touch him. He's doing fine." Tentatively touching her son, his mother followed the nurse's lead, "You are doing fine." His father kept repeating, "I love you, son."

Looking to the nurse for reassurance, his mother asked, "Can he hear us?" "Yes, he hears you," she replied as she refocused on her vigilant management of the patient's care. She touched his foot as she walked around his bed. As the family left, the nurse briefly turned from the patient to reassure them, "I'll take good care of him and call you with any change. Try to get some rest." She then received new blood gases and triumphantly held them to the door for his parents and the pulmonary fellow to see while reporting to the patient, "Your blood gases are great. You're doing very well."

At home with herself, the environment, and the patient, this nurse demonstrated nurse presence. She not only expertly managed the multiple demands of physical care but also was receptive to the emotional and psychological needs of her patient and his family. Indeed, she was attuned to such an extent that she recognized the ordinary effort of moving his foot from the covers as a signal that he was too warm. Respecting and responding to common human experiences like physical pain, unrealized hope, fear of the unknown, or being too warm, her presence enabled everyone to feel less isolated and afraid in the newness of the long-anticipated transplant.

Recognizing that nursing is a response to the full range of human experiences, Paterson and Zderad proposed that nurse presence requires openness, receptivity, and availability by the nurse to the manifold expressions of human experience. These writers noted that presence not only insists on "being at the other's disposal but also being with him with the whole of oneself" (Paterson & Zderad, 1988, p. 28). This is no small feat given the prerequisites of self-awareness, authenticity, courage, focused attention, and the choice to set aside for the moment the nurse's own needs for control to receive whatever the patient is experiencing.

This chapter highlights three features of presence:
- The practice of presence
- Telling the truth
- Presence and hope

The Practice of Presence

Human experiences can be imagined along on a continuum at one end of which is alienation and isolation while at the other is a full sense of connection with oneself, others, or a higher being (Younger, 1995). Alienation, or a sense of disconnection from oneself and others, leads to feelings of meaninglessness, powerlessness, loneliness, and loss of community, whereas connection brings a sense of unity with self and others and the feeling of "being a part of something that is greater than ourselves" (Younger, 1995, p. 60). The experience of suffering is isolating. Nurse presence enables a human connection and thus ends the isolation and brings meaning to the suffering.

Presence, or opening oneself to another, is perhaps the highest level of human caring. Beginning with the choice to set aside one's own needs for the moment, especially the need for control and certainty, nurse presence requires entering the experience of the patient with all of the uncertainty and surprise of such an endeavor. Presence requires exquisite and focused attention to the moment—noticing a foot slipping from the covers, a trembling hand, a single tear, the radiance of new parents, the gratitude for good news—and being open to join the patient in these experiences. Entering the patient's experience may involve listening, touching, feeling close, or attentively giving physical care (Benner, 1984; Doona, Haggerty, & Chase, 1997; Paterson & Zderad, 1988). Regardless of its form, nurse presence mitigates the isolation of suffering and joins the nurse and patient as fellows in the human experience.

The presence of the nurse depends upon both patient and nurse receptivity. Alert patients may signal receptivity to the nurse by verbal or nonverbal expressions of emotional vulnerability—for example, the mother of the young lung transplant patient said, "I am afraid." The unconscious patient or the very ill patient who cannot talk, like the young transplant patient described earlier, invites the caring presence of the nurse by his extreme vulnerability, which calls from the nurse protective and caring responses (Doona et al., 1997).

The nurse's receptivity to the patient begins with attention to the sometimes subtle and ordinary expressions of human experience: a stifled sob, the joy and amazement of a young couple giving birth, the slight turn of a woman's head away from her mastectomy wound, the shame of incontinence, the sigh of relief from pain. The receptive nurse notices these events and is drawn to the patient, turning to the patient to ask about her sob, quietly honoring the young couple's surprise and delight, gently touching the turned cheek of the woman who has lost her breast, reassuring the incontinent patient that she knows it is hard, or taking the hand of the patient in pain. No encounter with patients holds greater possibility for a creative expression of the best of the nurse than those occasions that elicit the nurse's presence. The form of nurse presence, directed by patient need, arises from the fully attentive nurse who is attuned to both herself and to her patient (Doona et al., 1997). Thus, nurse presence occasions growth for the nurse as a human being and as a professional whose role is fully realized in being present to the patient (Doona et al., 1997).

In an analysis of nurse interactions with ventilator-dependent, chronically ill patients, four levels of nurse presence have been described (Osterman & Schwartz-Barcott, 1996). At one level, the nurse is "physically present" in the patient's room but absorbed in her own thoughts, overlooking the patient. There is no interaction with the patient. This level of presence may occur when a novice nurse who is afraid of the equipment becomes preoccupied with her fears and fails to notice the patient's needs. A second level of presence occurs when the nurse is "partially present"; she initially notices and greets the patient but then goes about the tasks at hand without further attention to the patient. This level of nurse presence does not allow for connection with the patient but may reduce stress for the patient since the nurse is at least performing tasks on the patient's behalf.

"Full presence" occurs when the nurse engages with the patient in an empathetic, caring, receptive interaction that is directed toward meeting all the patient's needs. The nurse is attentive, listening, and focused on the here and now. Finally, "transcendent presence" entails an interaction between two people that is peaceful, comforting, transformative, and harmonious. Full presence diminishes the patient's loneliness and infuses the patient with a sense of hope and meaning. There is a connection in which the nurse feels "oneness with the patient," and both nurse and patient are transformed by an "energy that goes beyond the two people interacting" (Osterman & Schwartz-Barcott, 1996, p. 28).

Telling the Truth

In his book, *How We Die*, surgeon Sherwin Nuland described his wish to balance his dying brother's longing for cure with the reality of his terminal illness. Nuland recalled his failure to "speak the words that should have been said; I couldn't tolerate the immediate burden of hurting him, and so I exchanged the possibility of the comfort that may come with an unhampered death for the misconceived 'hope' that I thought I was giving him" (1994, p. 227). Nuland's efforts to protect his brother by giving him the hope for a cure in the face of widely metastatic cancer constituted a deception that became a source of added anguish for all as the dying brother was further isolated and underwent toxic chemotherapy to no avail. Had Nuland spoken the truth to his brother, he could have confronted the isolation of his own and his brother's suffering.

An essential aspect of nurse presence is telling patients the truth in a timely manner and remaining truthful as patients' experiences change in response to treatment and illness. Telling the truth is a finely developed art that begins with the recognition that the truth is not known by the nurse and brought to patients like nurses deliver medicine or treatments (Gadow, 1985). Medical facts can be told to patients, but the truth for patients is much richer and more complex than the medical facts. The truth for a patient evolves from the patient's circumstances, depends upon the patient's perception of what is going on, and changes as the patient's circumstances change. For example, in the vignette presented earlier, the medical facts indicated that the patient was doing well, yet for the mother, whose hopes and fears for her son prevented her from recognizing this, the truth was that she was afraid her son would die. The nurse responded to her fears, at the same time giving her the medical facts she needed to begin to temper those fears with a realistic picture of her son's condition. Telling the truth enables the nurse and patient to come to new understandings about what is true for the patient as the illness unfolds.

Most nurses and physicians agree that patients should be told the truth about their medical condition so that they will have an opportunity to modulate their expectations accordingly (Miller, 1991). But often patients and nurses do not share the same perceptions and beliefs about what constitutes medical reality (Stephenson, 1991). Even when patients hear the medical facts, they may still perceive the situation differently from nurses and doctors. For example, patients may give themselves the benefit of the doubt medically and downplay negative aspects of their condition. This may appear to be a form of denial or a distortion of the facts—and indeed, that may be the case. In some situations patients may frankly distort medical facts, leading to a failure to receive medical treatment or to put their affairs in order before dying. Nevertheless, these false or unrealistic perceptions may be useful to patients by providing them time to develop the coping skills needed to deal realistically with their illness.

There is no clear formula to guide the nurse in dealing with patients who refuse to accept the medical reality of their illness. Many nurses believe that the patient's perception of reality should be honored, whether this is consistent with the facts or not (Stephenson, 1991; Klyma & Vehvilainen-Julkunen, 1997). However, the distinction must be made between respecting a patient's *perception* of the medical reality and misleading the patient with false hopes or inaccurate or incomplete information. Others suggest that the nurse should continually help the patient see reality since there may be adverse consequences to a failure to do so (Yates, 1993). This effort is complicated by the temptation to give the patient false hope, not to protect the patient, but to protect the nurse from facing the patient's painful reality. This was demonstrated in the preceding account by Nuland (1994) of his brother's death. Ideally, the nurse maintains an equilibrium between these two extremes by her presence, enabling her to recognize and respond to the patient's perceptions while giving her a realistic picture of the medical realities.

Presence and Hope

Hope is a basic human response that gives meaning to life. Hope involves being open to future possibilities that arise from the present while being linked to the past. Hope is thus dynamic; while giving meaning to life and offering a means for coping with uncertainty (Miller, 1997), it changes in degree and focus over time (Kylma & Vehvilainen-Julkunen, 1997).

The presence of the nurse, coupled with telling the truth, is a major means for inspiring realistic hope in patients (Cutcliffe, 1995). That is because the presence of another person serves as a reminder of the wide range of human possibilities and responses in any given situation. Furthermore, the presence of the nurse provides comfort and support for the often painful feature of facing medical truths about illness.

Patients report that nurses influence their hope by taking time to talk, answering questions honestly, offering helpful information and listening to their concerns (Post-White et al., 1996). As patient realities shift, nurse presence helps patients realistically reformulate goals and hopes (Yates, 1993). Thus the presence and truthfulness of the nurse provide an anchor that helps patients maintain realistic hope to move toward health and recovery: when the situation is grim, nurse presence provides connection and thus relief from despair.

Hope has a strong affective, or feeling, component (Dufault & Martocchio, 1985). The feelings associated with hope include expectancy as well as the dynamic tension between hope and despair. While hope enables a patient to hold at bay feelings of despair, if hope is not realized, the patient may feel disappointment and even hopelessness. The presence of the nurse is key in helping the patient remain open to possibilities while focusing on the present moment since "the here and now is the only place and time we can be in, the only place and time we can effect change, and the only place and time we can appreciate life for what it is" (Greenhut, 1995, p. 27).

The story that follows is about the nurse's presence in response to the patient, Stan, and his wife, Helen. Edith cared for this couple through a short but intense illness during which their experience evolved from the hope for a cure to the expectation of a loving and supportive dying for Stan.

Edith's Story

Edith was a home health nurse, working in a hospice program. The day she received the referral for Stan's care and read his medical history, she thought, This one's going to be trouble for me. The patient was a young man with metastatic carcinoma. He was close to her age. Her husband had undergone successful treatment for cancer a year earlier, and she knew that her immediate identification with this patient meant she would be emotionally challenged by his care.

The patient, Stan, was a scientist whose cancer had been diagnosed three months earlier when tests revealed an abdominal tumor. The surgery was extensive, and the surgeon thought he got it all. Then, a few months later recurrent cancer invaded his abdomen and liver. Because the cancer returned quickly and extensively, Stan's prognosis was grim. Upon the rediscovery of cancer, he returned to the hospital for chemotherapy. The home health referral was for continuation of treatment at home.

Arriving at Stan's home for the first time, Edith found a healthy-looking, handsome outdoorsman and his wife, Helen, a loving and sprightly woman. A hospital bed was next to the couple's bed. On the wall was a colorful array of cutouts of individual hands, strung together with bright yarn. Earlier when Stan had been hospitalized for chemotherapy, Helen had taken construction paper, yarn, and scissors to the hospital and invited each individual who helped Stan, including physicians, nurses, housekeepers, and persons who delivered meal trays, to outline his hand and cut it out. Individuals signed the cutout and many wrote good wishes. Helen hung the "helping hands" on the wall in the hospital and now they adorned the bedroom at home, providing a reminder of the many people who helped Stan and creating a sense of being surrounded by love.

Stan was feeling reasonably well on this first visit. Edith, Helen, and Stan discussed his chemotherapy. Edith noted that Stan and Helen were aware of his grave prognosis but planned to continue treating the cancer aggressively, hoping for a cure. Edith did the necessary teaching about treatments, worked out the plan of care, and reassured the couple that they were all in this together for the long haul.

Returning to her car, Edith began to cry. Never before had she cried after an admission. She recalled her personal experience with cancer in her family, highlighted now by her recent meeting with Stan and Helen. Edith recognized that her identification with Stan and Helen was great, and this could compromise her care because she might be more focused on her own concerns than on those of the patient. She also knew that it could increase her sensitivity to Stan and Helen's needs because of their shared experience, strengthening her ability to help this couple. "The trick," Edith said, "was balancing these two possibilities. I felt I needed to talk this over with a colleague."

The next day Edith called a fellow nurse and they talked. As Edith shared her concerns related to caring for this couple, she received the support she needed and experienced a great release. "Talking to my friend and colleague was crucial to my ability to care for this family. Talking it out helped me consciously recognize the differences between my own experience with cancer in my family and the events Stan and Helen were enduring." After the call, having reestablished the distinctions and similarities between herself and the patient, Edith felt ready for the challenge and moved forward with the plan of care for Stan.

Initially Edith visited Stan three times a week, administering the complex chemotherapy while assessing Stan and Helen's response to the process. Managing the chemotherapy required great skill. Stan did not have a central line through which Edith could give his chemotherapy, so at each visit Edith had to start an intravenous line (IV) and administer Stan's medication, which was caustic and could cause tissue damage if it leaked from the vein. She also administered subcutaneous medications, assessed Stan's reaction to the chemotherapy, his pain level, and his ability to tolerate food and fluid.

Noting that Helen wanted to help with Stan's care, Edith taught her how to monitor Stan's fluid intake and his output and how to give the treatment that was administered through subcutaneous injections. She then supervised Helen until she mastered the skills. She also observed that Stan often refused to take medication for pain. Edith wondered if he associated the need for pain medications with the progression of his cancer. Edith observed that both Helen and Stan carefully recorded all the details of the chemotherapy, lab values, urine output, and fluid intake. Stan, who was less open with Edith than Helen, focused conversations almost exclusively on this recorded information, though Helen also talked about her fears and anxieties about Stan's illness. At each visit Edith made inquiries about how the family was coping. Learning that their two adolescent girls were having some difficulties in school and were experiencing more conflict with each other than usual, Edith made a referral to a nurse who specialized in working with adolescents and loss.

Despite aggressive chemotherapy, Stan's physical condition deteriorated rapidly. His weight dropped, his abdomen became distended, and Edith could easily feel the growing tumor. Edith drew a weekly sample of Stan's blood to keep apace of his blood profile. After each visit she called the physician to report the lab values. She also kept the physician abreast of Stan's decreasing tolerance of the toxic chemotherapy. She continued to share with Stan and Helen the lab findings, which reflected plummeting blood counts and aggressive tumor growth.

"We were doing all we could for Stan," said Edith, "and his condition was deteriorating steadily. I was pretty frustrated with his physician, who, despite the evidence of Stan's rapid decline, would not talk with them about the apparent failure of the chemotherapy. He just couldn't face it himself, I suppose. I kept telling him that the chemotherapy was going to kill Stan, and he could see that was true from Stan's poor lab values. Eventually the physician recommended that Stan 'take a rest' from the toxic treatment, explaining that Stan's extremely low blood counts made further treatment unsafe. I guess that was as direct as he could be," Edith concluded.

Even though Stan and Helen agreed to discontinue the chemotherapy for a while, Edith noted that they continued to talk about hope for recovery. Yet while they spoke about "getting a cure," Edith also noted cues that led her to believe they were reassessing their hope for a cure. For example, Stan began to admit that he was hurting and became more willing to take pain medication. The fact that it was becoming increasingly difficult for him to get out of bed to go to the bathroom could not be denied. Helen, previously intent on a precise administration of Stan's chemotherapy and related treatment medications, missed a dose one day. Most significantly, they stopped asking about the lab values.

Although Edith and the physician agreed that Stan was doing poorly and could not tolerate further treatment, the physician continued to avoid talking to Stan and Helen about Stan's declining physical status. Edith, however, felt compelled to talk with the couple. "I needed to get some idea of whether their perceptions of Stan's physical condition were realistic and to share with them what I was seeing. A patient cannot deal realistically with the situation without having a reasonable picture of the medical facts." Edith continued, "I knew that when patients are not able to hear the medical truth, they simply don't hear it. With defense mechanisms in place, they continue to deny what they have been told. But I had to assess what Stan and Helen were thinking. I knew from the changes in their behavior that at a deep level they knew things were not going well for Stan."

With this in mind, Edith decided to talk with Stan and Helen. This was not unfamiliar territory for Edith. It would be a hard talk because Edith knew it would be painful for Stan and Helen. She explained, "I believed it was better for them to cry over the truth than for them to know in their hearts that things were not going well and to dishonor that by ignoring it and hence live and die a lie. I knew from past experience that if they could hear me, the very act of telling them the truth could provide the occasion for our sharing this painful reality and we would all be less isolated."

Shortly after the treatments were discontinued, Edith approached Stan and Helen to ask how they felt things were going. She heard in their response their questioning of Stan's progress. She told them what she had observed and what she knew—that Stan was not doing well, at present he could not tolerate any more chemotherapy, and it did not look good for him. Edith did not directly address the fact that Stan was dying. Indeed, she listened to their perceptions and answered their questions, giving them evidence of the progression of Stan's disease, thus providing the facts they needed to begin to confront their ebbing hope for a cure.

Shortly after this, Helen admitted Stan to the hospital, explaining that she couldn't bear to see him waste away. He received a blood transfusion and went home. No one in the hospital spoke to Stan and Helen of his rapidly failing physical condition. The transfusion perked Stan up a bit and, then, for the first time, he spoke openly with Edith about concerns other than the treatment. One day as she cared for Stan he said, "I hope I can make it for two more weeks. My daughter is going to receive a special recognition at her school."

"Yes, I share that hope," Edith responded, noting that Stan had made a notable shift away from the belief that he could be cured. This statement was grounded in the reality of his declining physical state and in his love for his daughter. After this conversation Edith noted, "Stan had referred indirectly to his own death. I now knew that he was aware he was dying. I felt relief for myself and for him, since he could deal realistically with what was happening to him and his family." To help him keep up with the passing days until his daughter's special event, Edith placed a calendar by his bed. Together, Stan and Helen marked the days until the day of recognition arrived for his daughter, who proudly showed her father her award.

The Christmas holidays were approaching. Edith had a two-week vacation coming up. Edith said, "I needed some time off. My two teenage daughters needed time with me, and our family deserved quality time without interruptions by my work. So with a heavy heart I turned the care of this family over to another nurse for two weeks. I hated to leave them during this time, and in a way I betrayed them by doing so since they leaned heavily upon me. But I have learned that there are limits to what I can do as a nurse, and I have to take care of myself so that I can care for my patients."

About a week before her vacation, Edith told Helen and Stan that she would be gone for two weeks. They received the news with disappointment and dismay. Edith requested that one of her colleagues, whom she knew to be an excellent nurse, take over the care of the family. Edith and the replacement nurse went together for a visit so that Edith could show her all the details about Stan's care. Before they left, the two nurses sat with Helen over a cup of coffee while they talked about the family's needs.

Edith urged Helen to observe Christmas fully that year. Stan's family was coming, Helen said, as well as her own. Helen had already arranged for the couple's pastor, along with the extended family, to celebrate a candlelight service in their home on Christmas Eve.

As it turned out, Christmas was a bittersweet time for Helen, Stan, and the girls. They all knew that it would be their last Christmas as a family. The Christmas Eve service was the highlight for Helen. "The memory of the loveliness of the candlelight upon the faces of the family members will always stay with me. It was deeply moving," Helen said later to Edith.

Edith returned to her care of the family shortly after Christmas. Stan was much weaker, but Helen was still reluctant to face his impending death. Days before Stan died and longing to protect him from his impending death, Helen once again took Stan to the hospital. Reflecting on this, Edith observed, "Helen took him to the hospital because he was so weak and she wanted to do something. She also needed to talk to a doctor, just to be sure there was nothing else to be done for Stan. The doctor remained reluctant to talk with them about Stan's situation. But he did agree to hospitalize Stan one last time."

During this hospitalization a physician consultant was called. He had not previously worked with the couple, but he told them directly: "Stan is within days of death and there is nothing we can do. Let's get you home while we can." Sobbing, her last hope gone, Helen called Edith for comfort. Edith listened as Helen's grief poured out. As the conversation ended, Helen said, "Let's get on with what we need to do for Stan."

Edith recalled, "I was amazed at Helen's bravery. Her heart was broken, but she was able to shift her focus rapidly away from her grief to Stan's needs. That was a hard phone call for me. I had grown attached to this couple, and I was very sad."

Helen expressed her determination and hope to make this experience a good one for Stan. Edith recalled, "We were now united in our efforts to address Stan's suffering and make him feel loved and secure during his time of dying."

When Stan returned home, Edith was waiting with an order for morphine for his pain. Stan had come from the hospital with an intravenous line (IV) in place to provide him fluid. He was too weak to drink. Since everyone knew that Stan was now at home to die, Edith discussed with the couple the possibility of removing the IV. She explained that the IV would prolong his dying and that without an IV, Stan would not suffer from thirst since thirst is a function of living, not dying. Helen interrupted, "I want him to have the IV. It represents a way that we can help Stan." The IV remained in place. Edith recognized, "The IV was there to help Helen, not Stan. This was hard for me to accept. Helen felt better with the IV in place, and Stan felt better because Helen was comforted by the IV, so I guess you could say that indirectly his needs were met. However, from my perspective, his physical needs would have been better served if we had discontinued the IV. Frankly, I was not sure what to do, and I still don't know whether I did what was best for Stan."

The next day the IV became occluded, and it needed to be restarted. Edith said to Stan and Helen, "Do you want to reinsert this? It is up to you."

Stan replied, "Whatever Helen wants." Helen's response was quick, "I want him to have it."

As Edith prepared to restart the IV, she noticed Stan crying. Edith was taken aback when he explained, "I'm scared, I'm afraid of what you are about to do to me."

Profoundly touched by this expression of fear and Stan's sharing of his vulnerable and deeply human nature with her, Edith replied, "I am so sorry to have to hurt you. Do you still want the IV?"

Stan nodded yes, and reluctantly she restarted the IV, recognizing that this met Helen's need to do something for Stan and Stan's wish to honor Helen's request. Fortunately, the IV went in without difficulty.

During the last days of Stan's life he was mostly unresponsive, his pulse thready. Helen moved toward acceptance of his approaching death. She was able to say to Edith, "I am at peace with this." Helen remained at Stan's bedside, joined now by the children, the extended family, and her best friend. Edith visited daily. On these occasions she involved herself with those in attendance, talking with them about their common past and helping them look toward a shared future without Stan. There was a sense of closeness as the women in the family joined Edith in providing Stan's care.

Several days before Stan's death, Helen showed Edith a beautiful unlit candle beside Stan's bed. An intensely spiritual couple, Helen explained, "I will light the candle after Stan dies as a way of saying good-bye to his spirit."

Stan lingered for another day, then died peacefully, surrounded by his family. After his death, Helen called Edith, who arrived to find the extended family with Helen and the children in the bedroom. Stan was lying in the hospital bed, his arms crossed, the candle burning, and the priest saying prayers with the family. When the ritual was completed, Edith pronounced him dead and took out the dreaded IV. Helen accompanied the body outside to the waiting hearse.

Two days later Edith attended the funeral. "I don't usually go to the patient's funeral, but sometimes I need that ritual to say good-bye. This couple had touched me and I wanted to honor them and my work with them. So I went to the service."

During the service, on the occasion of the passing of the peace, Helen asked Edith to come and join the family for the remainder of the service. Edith wept with Helen, the children, and Stan's extended family. She explained, "I think the family asked me to join them because they had experienced me as a real person. I engaged with them with all that I am, with all of my life experiences, not just in a role of nurse. I was a real person who cried and could agree that this was a terrible situation. I could say I was sorry when I had to hurt Stan, rather than keeping him at some clinical distance. It is a fearful thing to take someone into your home to die—the patriarch, the father, the husband, the lover—and you need someone there to say, 'This is OK, this will be OK.' . . . And it was."

Enacting Artful Nursing

This discussion focuses on four nursing actions as they are highlighted in Edith's story:
- Nurse presence
- Telling the truth
- Establishing trust
- Collaboration

NURSE PRESENCE

Stan was referred to the home health agency to continue his chemotherapy treatments. The primary nursing task was to administer the chemotherapy and assess Stan's responses to the treatment. However, from the outset Edith regarded her work with Stan and Helen as much more than the administration of chemotherapy. Edith explained, "I was engaged with them with all that I was. I was not simply a nurse who did treatments but I also related to them as a mother, a wife, and caretaker." Edith described this as being "present" to the couple.

For Edith, being present entailed being available and receptive to the family experience. She did not turn away when the news was bad but stepped up her engagement by speaking more directly of Stan's deteriorating medical situation and joining Helen in making Stan's dying peaceful. Further, she did not focus on nursing tasks alone. She did not see Stan as simply a disease to be treated and did not see herself simply as a nurse who treated disease. Rather, Edith offered herself as a whole person when she inquired about the children, recognized Helen's need to learn how to care for Stan, and affirmed Helen's fears and Stan's hope to live to see his daughter honored. This presence enabled Edith to recognize the importance of Helen's sadness and fear, the couple's concern for the children's well-being, the supportive role of Helen's friends, the family's shared love, the significance of celebrating the last Christmas together, and Stan's wish to live to see his daughter recognized.

Edith brought to her care of the family her knowledge of many aspects of human experiences, including what it means to have a loved one diagnosed with cancer. She was able to recognize and respond to a multitude of matters beyond the importance of Stan's treatment and could observe with satisfaction, "I think the family . . . experienced me as a real person. I engaged with them with all that I am, with all of my life experiences, not just in a role of nurse. I was a real person who cried and could agree that this was a terrible situation. I could say I was sorry when I had to hurt Stan rather than keeping him at some clinical distance."

Self-reflection is a means of learning about oneself from nurse-patient encounters. Self-reflection is a prerequisite for the presence of the nurse since self-awareness, coupled with sensitivity to the patient, guides genuine encounters with the patient. Self-reflection is the process of self-examination and self-awareness in which the nurse, before entering into a helping relationship, examines her own needs, particularly as they might interfere with her ability to help the patient. Cutcliffe (1995) describes this as "reflection in action." Self-reflection was evident when, shortly after her initial encounter with Stan and Helen, Edith began to cry. Recognizing her strong identification with the couple's situation, she wisely called a colleague for support. The comfort she received helped her remember her distinctiveness from the patient and freed her to focus on Stan and Helen's needs rather than her own. It also helped her recognize how the similarities of their experiences would strengthen her empathic response to the family. Her identification with this family was then appropriately used to convey a sense of shared experience rather than lead to overidentification, thus jeopardizing her ability to provide excellent care. No longer impeded by overidentifying with the couple, Edith could join them in their experience and declare, "We are in this together for the long haul."

Self-reflection was also evident in Edith's recognition of her ambivalence about leaving Stan and Helen during her vacation and the possible betrayal of her patient this represented. Edith had learned that "there are limits to what I can do as a nurse, and I have to take care of myself so that I can care for my patients." Rather than ignore her feelings about separating from the family when they needed her, Edith took note of her concerns and duly arranged excellent care for Stan, orientation for the new nurse, and time for the transition to a new caregiver.

TELLING THE TRUTH

It is easy for the nurse to offer false hope to patients, but telling the truth is essential to helping patients establish hope for what is attainable. In this narrative, telling the truth was key to helping Stan and Helen focus on hopes beyond cure, such as Stan's hope to see his daughter honored and Edith's hope for a peaceful dying for Stan. Other patients might hope to set right broken relationships, get business affairs in order, live until the birth of an expected grandchild, or finish a writing project. Without some truth about the medical condition, however, patients may not be able to envision realistic hopes.

Early in their experience of Stan's illness, the truth for Stan and Helen was that a cure was possible, and their hopes arose from this. As Stan's condition deteriorated, it was no longer true that Stan could be cured. But for the couple, who had not yet consciously recognized Stan's declining state, the truth was that there was still realistic hope for cure. This hope was not based on medical reality but it grew out of the couple's perception of the truth at the time: they had had little chance to get used to the idea of Stan's death, their teenage girls needed the guidance of their father, Stan was young and only months before had been vigorous, and Helen could not yet imagine herself without her husband. All of these contingencies conspired to support their hope for a cure, even in the face of Stan's declining condition.

Recognizing the complexity of the truth for this couple, Edith did not set out to supplant their "unrealistic" truth with a medical version of what was true. She focused on leaving open possibilities for this couple while also steering them away from what was clearly impossible—a cure for Stan. Tuned into their experience, she noted cues indicating their changing perceptions, such as Helen missing a medication and Stan's diminishing interest in his lab values. She talked with them about the situation and invited the couple to look with her at what was happening. She asked what they were thinking and feeling about Stan's treatment. She gave them information about Stan's decline. She helped them incorporate medical truths into their ever-changing perceptions of what was happening to Stan and to their family. This process was accelerated when the physician consultant told the couple that Stan had only days to live. At this point, Edith's supportive presence enabled Helen to put aside her fears and declare, "Let's get on with what we need to do for Stan."

ESTABLISHING TRUST

As the nurse demonstrates sensitivity and receptivity to the patient's experience, trust develops, which in turn enables continued self-expression by the patient and the nurse. Trust in Edith began for Stan and Helen when they noted her competence in managing Stan's complex treatment. Indeed, competence in implementing basic and complex skills is fundamental to all aspects of artful nursing and most patients trust the nurse's competence. The competent nurse who shows—as Edith did—a compassionate and supportive response to the patient, however, earns a greater trust. This trust was reinforced for Stan and Helen when Edith assured them that she would be there for the long haul and the couple learned they could count on Edith.

Edith also trusted Stan and Helen. This trust emboldened her to speak truthfully about the progression of Stan's disease. And the couple's trust in Edith sustained their ability to gradually hear the meaning of Edith's painful words. Reciprocal trust sustained this threesome and helped set the stage for a rich and meaningful experience for everyone. Fortunately, the trust between Edith and the couple was not ruptured by Edith's vacation, which came at a time when the couple needed Edith. Stan and Helen's trust in Edith could have ended when she left them at this point. Edith's sensitivity to this possibility guided her careful preparation for her departure, including preparing the couple, requesting a well-respected and competent colleague to take over the care, and thoroughly orienting the new nurse to the family.

COLLABORATION

A second expression of the mutual trust between Edith, Stan, and Helen was evident in their collaborative efforts. As collaborators, the couple and Edith were all engaged in Stan's care. Collaboration supports a partnership between the nurse and patient in which the nurse trusts the patient, the patient trusts the nurse, and care is negotiated rather than imposed. The consequence of this for patients like Stan and Helen is that they gain some control and an affirmation of their self-knowledge (Cutcliffe, 1995). For the nurse, collaboration offers the opportunity to learn from the patient and provide individualized care.

Recognizing the couple as collaborators, Edith carefully responded to what they said and to unspoken cues, particularly those cues indicating a recognition of Stan's declining physical condition. Collaboration between Edith and the couple required Edith's acknowledgment that Stan and Helen were capable of participating in their care and knew many of their needs better than Helen. They knew how long they needed to monitor Stan's lab values carefully and when they were ready to loosen their focus on this objective measure of his status. Helen took her cues in these matters from the couple.

Collaboration occurred when Stan and Helen participated in treatment decisions and closely followed Stan's lab values. Helen initiated two brief hospitalizations for palliative care and helped administer Stan's chemotherapy. During Stan's last days, it would have been easy for Edith simply to recommend discontinuation of the IV. However, she turned to Stan and Helen to determine their wishes regarding the discontinuation of Stan's IV. Recognizing the conflicting needs of Stan, Helen, and her own need to support Stan optimally in an uncomplicated dying, Edith navigated her way through the competing concerns, acknowledging her lack of clarity at this point with regard to the best course.

Challenges to Nurse Presence

There are individuals who cannot be receptive to the presence of the nurse and who do not desire the nurse's presence. There are also occasions when the presence of the nurse is not useful to the nurse or the patient. Efforts to engage a patient may increase patient anxiety, the patient may not want to be connected with the nurse, or the patient may feel overwhelmed and may not have the energy for engagement (Osterman & Schwartz-Barcott, 1996). The receptive nurse will note these occasions and respect the patient's needs.

Perhaps the most pressing challenge to nursing efforts to be present to patients is nurse burnout. (See Chapter 10 for a full discussion of burnout.) Feelings of overextension by nurses lead to indifference toward patients and a focus on nursing tasks at the expense of responding to less evident patient needs. Given the complexity of patient care and the unrelenting nature of patient need, there are times when burnout is inevitable. At other times the nurse may have personal concerns or an excessive workload that requires most of the nurse's energy, leaving only enough time or endurance to give technically competent care. During these times, self-reflection enables the nurse to recognize encroaching indifference toward patients and to take self-sustaining action. Engagement with patients at the level of nursing tasks alone is not satisfying to either patient or nurse. Nurse self-reflection and self-sustaining behaviors are critical to counter burnout and to enable the nurse to be present to the patient.

Self-reflection, a corequisite to meaningful nurse-patient encounters, requires skill and insight along with continuing assessment of one's feelings and responses to patient circumstances and behavior. This requires time and is rarely easy in the busy and often hectic work environment. Self-reflection is greatly facilitated when the nurse has a sympathetic colleague with whom she can talk about feelings that arise in response to patients. Despite the challenges to self-reflection, in the long run self-reflection saves the nurse time and energy because it enables the nurse to distinguish between patient concerns and the concerns of the nurse, freeing the nurse to focus on the patient.

Central to presence with patients is telling the truth. There are, however, constraints on telling the truth to patients. In some institutions, the role of the nurse does not include giving patients any *new* medical information; the physician does this. Sometimes physicians wait to deliver unpleasant news until the patient feels better or, as in Stan's case, refuse to tell the hard truths. At other times family members try to protect patients from bad news, or communication simply breaks down, resulting in a delay in delivering new medical information to patients. Thus the nurse may have information that she is not free to deliver. In other situations, patients themselves wish not to be told the truth if the news is bad. And sometimes nurses join the conspiracy to conceal the truth of a poor medical prognosis from patients. Withholding the truth from patients is most often motivated by what is perceived to be the best interest of the patient. There are, however, few moral justifications for withholding from patients the truth about their condition, even though it is painful to give or receive this kind of information.

Trust in the nurse is encouraged by genuine nurse-patient encounters and by nurse competence. Building trust is not always easy. Some patients do not easily confer trust. Patient trust is influenced by many factors including the patient's prior or present negative experiences with health care providers and the increasing climate of mistrust in an increasingly impersonal health care system. There are patients whose lack of engagement with the nurse makes it difficult to work with them as trusted partners in their care. Nevertheless, the nurse has a responsibility to be trustworthy, given the vulnerability of patients and the assumption by most that the nurse will protect them from harm.

Collaboration, an outgrowth of trust and nurse presence, may also present great challenges to the nurse. In many cases it is quicker and easier to make decisions for the patient and exclude them from collaborative endeavors. In other situations, collaboration is stifled by patients who are not willing or able to be partners in their care. Some are too ill, others have never acted on their own behalf, and still others cannot overcome the intimidation of the health care system and express their needs. Nevertheless, the artful nurse approaches all patients, as Edith did, with an attitude that bolsters collaboration in their nursing care.

Summary

The presence of the nurse is perhaps the highest expression of care. Nurse presence ruptures the alienation and isolation of suffering and confirms joyful celebrations of human experience. A central feature of nurse presence is telling the truth and offering a realistic picture of the patient's medical situation. Presence, along with telling the truth, enables the establishment of realistic hopes by providing a supportive and realistic context for patient coping. Key nursing actions that support nursing presence include self-reflection, telling the truth, building trust, and nurse-patient collaboration. Despite the many obstacles to nursing presence, this is an essential feature of dealing with illness, recovery, or death.

References

Benner, P. (1984). *From novice to expert*. Menlo Park, CA: Addison-Wesley.

Cutcliffe, J.R. (1995). How do nurses inspire and instill hope in terminally ill HIV patients? *Journal of Advanced Nursing, 22*, 888–895.

Doona, M.E., Haggerty, L.A., & Chase, S.K. (1997). Nursing presence: An existential exploration of the concept. *Scholarly Inquiry for Nursing Practice, 11*, 3–16.

Dufault, K., & Martocchio, B.C. (1985). Hope: Its spheres and dimensions. *Nursing Clinics of North America, 20*, 379–391.

Gadow, S.A. (1985). Nurse and patient: The caring relationship. In A.H. Bishop & J.R. Scudder (Eds.), *Caring, curing and coping*. Birmingham: University of Alabama Press.

Greenhut, J.H. (1995). Living without hope. *Second Opinion, 21*, 27–33.

Kylma, J., & Vehvilainen-Julkunen, K. (1997). Hope in nursing research: A meta-analysis of the ontological and epistemological foundations of research on hope. *Journal of Advanced Nursing, 25*, 364–371.

Miller, B.K., Haber, J., & Byrne, M.W. (1992). The experience of caring in the acute care setting: Patient and nurse perspective. In D.A. Gaut (Ed.), *The presence of caring in nursing*. New York: National League for Nursing Press.

Miller, C.M. (1997). The lived experience of relapsing multiple sclerosis: A phenomenological study. *Journal of Neuroscience Nursing, 29*, 294–304.

Miller, J.F. (1991). Developing and maintaining hope in families of the critically ill. *AACN Clinical Issues in Critical Care, 2*, 307–315.

Nuland, S.B. (1994). *How we die*. New York: Alfred A. Knopf.

Ostermann, P., & Schwartz-Barcott, D. (1996). Presence: Four ways of being there. *Nursing Forum, 31*(2), 23–30.

Paterson, J.G., & Zderad, L.T. (1988). *Humanistic nursing*. New York: National League for Nursing Press.

Post-White, J., Ceronsky, C., Kreitzer, M.J., Nickelson, K., Drew, D., Mackey, K.W., Koopmeiners, L., & Gutknecht, S. (1996). Hope, spirituality, sense of coherence, and quality of life in patients with cancer. *Oncology Nursing Forum, 23*, 1571–1579.

Stephenson, C. (1991). The concept of hope revisited for nursing. *Journal of Advanced Nursing, 16*, 1456–1461.

Yates, P. (1993). Towards a reconceptualization of hope for patients with a diagnosis of cancer. *Journal of Advanced Nursing, 18*, 701–706.

Younger, J.B. (1995). The alienation of the sufferer. *Advances in Nursing Science, 17*(4), 53–72.

APPLICATION

....

ACTIVITY I
Group Discussion: Analysis of the Story

1. What do you think about Edith's decision to continue to care for Stan and Helen when, after her first visit, she recognized the possibility of overidentification with her patient? What would you have done and why? Discuss options other than the one Edith chose. To whom would you turn for support and guidance in such a situation?

2. What would you have done when Helen requested that Stan's IV, which was no longer medically necessary, be reinserted and Stan, fearful of the pain of the procedure, agreed to the IV to please Helen? What other approaches could Edith have taken with this couple?

3. How would you have responded to the physician who refused to be involved in telling the truth to Stan and Helen? What would your reasons be for this approach to the physician? What do you think were his reasons for failing to address the truth of Stan's declining medical situation?

4. Discuss the constraints to telling the truth that were evident in Edith's story. How would you confront those constraints?

5. What do you think about Edith's decision to attend Stan's funeral? Do you think the nurse should attend a patient's funeral? Defend your position.

ACTIVITY II
Self-Reflection: Experiencing Presence

Write about a time in your life when you have experienced the presence of a friend, or offered your presence to another person.

1. Paying attention to the details, describe what this experience was like for you.

2. Describe the positive and negative feelings you had when the experience was complete.

3. What did you learn from this experience that will be useful to you in your nursing practice?

ACTIVITY III
Self-Reflection: Assessing Personal Strengths

1. Draw a circle. Divide this circle into four pie-shaped segments, letting each segment represent one of the nursing actions described in this chapter: Nurse presence, telling the truth, establishing trust, and collaboration. Allocate size to each segment, making those segments representing an area in which you have greater strengths larger than the segments representing areas of your present limitations.

2. Examine your circle and consider which areas you need to develop as you grow in your nursing practice.

3. List three specific ways you can enhance your skills in the areas you identified as limitations.

ACTIVITY IV
Group Discussion: Assessing
Common Themes

1. Compare your pie-shaped circles. Which segments are larger? Smaller?

2. How do you explain any similarities or themes reflected in this group comparison?

3. Which of the themes present the greatest challenge to your group members and why?

4. How can nursing students help each other overcome these challenges? Be specific about ways you can help each other.

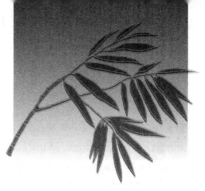

CHAPTER 10

Caring for Oneself

Introduction

The final chapter of this text focuses on self-care and is in many ways the most important of the book. Without self-care, the nurse will sooner or later succumb to feelings of chronic depletion, anger, resentment, and frustration, which jeopardize the well-being of both the nurse and the patient.

The challenge of caring for oneself in nursing is a mighty one and means dealing with multiple obstacles. Some barriers exist in all nursing specialties and care settings, while others are specific to particular settings. Impediments to self-care may be professional or system driven, for example, excessive workloads or ineffective management. Obstacles to self-care may also be personal, like unrealistic expectations for oneself. Despite the challenges to self-care, caring for oneself is central to effectively caring for others.

Self-care is care of the *self* in the deepest sense. It arises from a sense of self-worth and self-awareness, is unrelenting in the requirement of vigilance, and, like all skills in nursing, requires practice.

The chapter explores three factors that may affect self-care efforts of nurses:

- Burnout
- Professional dynamics
- Personal dynamics

Burnout

Nurses provide services around the clock in a wide variety of settings. In most of these settings, the individuals they care for are vulnerable and needy, and nurses' actions have a dramatic impact upon patient well-being. Given the scope and weight of nursing concerns, it is no surprise that burnout is a familiar experience for nurses (Duquette, Kerouac, Sandhu, & Beaudet, 1994). Nursing care is stressful, and in the rapidly changing health care system, few nurses are immune to feeling overwhelmed at times.

In order to confront nursing practice with responsible, proactive self-care responses, it is important to recognize the features of burnout. Burnout has been described as a depletion of personal resources resulting in physical, emotional, and cognitive exhaustion (Kushnir, Rabin, & Azulai, 1997). The nurse lacks energy, becomes irritable, anxious, and angry, and has feelings of helplessness and hopelessness. Physical manifestations may include headaches, backaches, or gastrointestinal disorders. Eventually the nurse develops negative attitudes and persistent feelings of coldness, cynicism, and indifference to patients. These feelings lead to a negative self-image, guilt, and a sense of personal failure; as a result, the nurse dreads going to work and feels increasingly guilty because of poor care of patients or indifference to them (Duquette et al., 1994; Farrington, 1997).

While a direct relationship has not been established between setting or type of patient and burnout (Duquette et al., 1994), many setting- and patient-related factors have been associated with burnout. For example, a demand for technological excellence, constant noise, and impending crises of patients and families—all high stress—characterize critical care units and contribute to burnout (Sawatzky, 1997). Bone marrow transplant units, where nurse-patient relationships are intense and treatment is life-threatening, are also high stress and may lead to burnout (Molassiotis & Haberman, 1996). There are stresses in caring for HIV-positive patients, many of whom live with stigma and fear, may die young, and, in addition, bring a risk of transmission of HIV to the nurse (Burr, 1996). Caring for critically ill pediatric patients is emotionally draining, especially when the child does not recover and experiences suffering that is difficult to relieve (Kennedy & Barloon, 1997).

Undergraduate nursing students experience burnout at levels comparable to those of working nurses (Haack, 1988). Students report feeling engulfed by school, work, family, and social demands; time pressures that prevent exercise and outlets for stress; physical complaints including debilitating fatigue; a feeling of being overwhelmed; poor concentration and motivation; and stressful relationships with families and friends (Beck, 1995).

One of Beck's (1995) respondents, describing her nursing school experience, said: "A month ago, I found myself facing a week with a patho exam, a pharmacology exam, a research paper, and I had to rewrite another paper which was due the same day as the other one. I was so overloaded with work I wanted to give up. I couldn't study anymore and I did bad[ly] on an exam because I just couldn't take it anymore. There was never a time when I could rest. . . . [There was no] way to relieve stress" (p. 22).

There are many ways to deal with burnout, ranging from attitudinal changes to finding a new work setting. Particular responses to burnout depend on the factors contributing to the burnout and the options available. However, certain commonly recognized antidotes to burnout may be useful to new nurses. For example, Vicenzi et al. (1997) suggest that feeling stressed and swamped by work can be altered by abandoning unrealistic notions of control, accepting the reality of change and the unpredictability of the future, continuing to learn new ways to do things, and joining forces with colleagues from related disciplines to adapt to the changes in health care.

Other strategies for confronting burnout include seeking support from colleagues or management. Duquette et al. (1994) note that "The more the nurse perceives receiving support in the workplace, the less he or she burns out" (p. 349). Support may take many forms, including rotating for several weeks to less stressful units, taking time off occasionally for oneself or for professional development, or participating in a multidisciplinary team to share decision making and responsibility for patients (Burr, 1996).

Professional Dynamics

Professional dynamics identified as challenges to artful nursing include heavy workloads, increasingly ill patients, growing demands for technological competence, institutional downsizing, ethical challenges, and a tension between the requirements of caring and those of an economically driven health care system. All of these factors challenge self-care efforts.

There are also aspects of the profession that threaten self-care. For example, nurses are expected to be caring, even when the system in which they work undermines and devalues the activities of care (Reverby, 1987). This catch-22 is rooted in nursing history. In the latter part of the nineteenth century when women had limited rights and almost all nurses were women, hospital administrators developed hospital-based nursing schools primarily to provide cheap student labor. Students were taught to follow orders, make few demands, and understand nursing as a duty with few accompanying rights. Altruism, sacrifice, and submission to others in power were expected, encouraged, and indeed, required. Thus, early in the development of the profession, nurses were led by social conditions and ideology to provide nursing care as an altruistic endeavor, to obey orders without question, and to abdicate claims to professional autonomy and rights (Reverby, 1987). This sociological and psychological framework set the stage for nurses to allow themselves to be submissive, obedient, and ultimately oppressed (Roberts, 1983); it effectively silenced the voice of nurses (Pike, 1997) and undermined self-care.

Many nurses still see themselves as "only a staff nurse" who just follows orders (Warner, Black, & Parent, 1998, p. 396), reinforcing the view that the nurse is powerless and oppressed. Further, the restructuring of health care, closing of nursing units and reduction of staff, coupled with the turmoil that accompanies change, "can quickly and insidiously lure articulate, autonomous professionals into the perceived safety of being but a cog in a bureaucratic wheel" (Pike, 1997, p. 532).

In the early 1980s, Roberts (1983) identified a major professional impediment to self-care: oppressed group behavior. Freire (1971), who observed the behavior of Brazilians who had been overtaken and dominated by Europeans, originally described this kind of behavior. Freire proposed that groups that are subordinate to more powerful groups in a society develop low self-esteem and self-hatred. This occurs because the dominant group establishes its own characteristics as most valuable, and the attributes of the subordinate group are considered inferior.

Roberts (1983) suggested that nurses, understanding their relationship to physicians as subordinate, have taken on the attributes of an oppressed group such as low self-esteem. This is evident in comments by nurses that undermine themselves or the profession such as, "It sure is hard to work with a bunch of women" or "I know this is a stupid question, but . . ." (Keen, 1990). Further, many nurses have identified with physicians and become dependent upon physicians for self-definition and support. These nurses tiptoe around advocacy efforts on behalf of patients, value compliments from physicians more than compliments from other nurses, and consider it flattering when someone says, "You are so smart, you should be a doctor" (Keen, 1991).

Roberts (1983) says that many nurses seek but never achieve full acceptance by the profession of medicine. Frustrated, these nurses become marginal and passive, ultimately succumbing to feelings of victimization, self-hatred, and dislike for other nurses and behaving in dependent, submissive, and passive-aggressive ways (McCall, 1996; Roberts, 1983, 1998). Noting that most nurses readily relate stories of oppression, McCall says that nurses may "adopt adaptive strategies of oppressed groups and direct their dissatisfaction inward toward each other, toward themselves and toward those less powerful than themselves" (p. 28). This phenomenon has been labeled "horizontal violence" (McCall, 1996), and it is seen when nurses squabble among themselves, take their frustrations out on other nurses, get angry at the profession for something that was not the profession's fault, or put down the profession when talking with other professionals (Keen, 1991).

Perhaps the greatest price of feeling oppressed and victimized is the failure of authenticity: nurses who succumb to these feelings are not true to themselves or to their profession. A failure of authenticity occurs, for example, when the nurse knows that a patient has not been fully informed about a procedure and does nothing, simply to avoid rocking the boat, or when the nurse practices on the assumption that nurses should always be caring and loving, denying the reality that nurses also get angry (Keen, 1991). Authenticity, or self-integrity, is key to self-care because authenticity supports feelings of self-worth and guides self-awareness. Self-worth and self-awareness in turn inform the nurse of self-care requirements. Without authenticity, nurses see themselves as victims of the changes in health care systems and succumb to powerlessness and hopelessness (Pike, 1997), rendering self-care impossible. However, when nurses seize opportunities for expression of the ideals of the profession through creativity, skill, and knowledge, they also elect a path of authenticity and self-care.

Personal Dynamics

Personal factors also affect self-care. Obviously, interpersonal, financial, physical, or psychological worries have an impact upon caring for oneself at work. Less obvious and therefore more threatening is a seductive feature of caring that potentially impedes the ability to care for anyone, including oneself. It has to do with the idea of self-sacrifice, a common pitfall for nurses (Caffey & Caffey, 1994).

It is easy to care for others at the expense of caring for oneself. Indeed, a popular stereotype of the ideal nurse is "one who *sacrifices* [italics added] her own needs to care for her patients, physicians, and the medical system itself" (Caffey & Caffey, 1994, p. 13). *Self-sacrifice* is incompatible with self-care. While nursing is hard work, nursing does not require the *sacrifice of the nurse herself*. (There are exceptions to this, obviously, as in wartime or emergency situations when the lives of both patients and nurses are threatened.)

The nurse is regularly required to make little sacrifices on behalf of patients, like postponing lunch to get a pain medication for a patient or staying late to help with an emergency. Occasionally, the nurse may have to come in to work on a day off. Determining the point at which sacrifice of the self occurs is an individual matter determined by the particulars of the situation. In general, however, self-sacrifice occurs when the demands of the job threaten the well-being of the nurse, for example, when the nurse is required for an *extended* period of time to work double shifts or to work on her days off. When excessive work demands leave no time or energy for oneself or one's other interests, the self is sacrificed to the work.

While self-sacrifice is not a requirement of the profession, it may be self-imposed, motivated by the need to feel appreciated, worthwhile, and competent (Caffey & Caffey, 1994). In situations where the nurse's need to be appreciated and desired drives the nurse's response, caring for others easily slips into self-sacrifice. A vicious cycle is then created. The nurse seeks acceptance and approval for her caring. When these are not forthcoming, the nurse feels unappreciated, angry, or ashamed. Motivated by fear of further rejection, failure, or conflict, the nurse tries even harder to gain acceptance (Caffey & Caffey, 1994). This vicious cycle excludes self-care and ultimately renders the nurse ineffective. For example, had Jana (in Chapter 5) depended upon the approval of her physician colleagues for her sense of well-being, she could not have advocated effectively for her patient Margaret.

When caring stems from a desire and intention to relieve human suffering rather than the nurse's need to be appreciated, the nurse does not require a particular response from the patient. Caring is experienced as "a spiritual bond between those involved in the caring relationship . . . [and] is an energizing phenomenon" (Caffey & Caffey, 1994, p. 15) for both nurse and patient. The nurse freely offers caring as a part of the nursing role because he desires to connect with and assist the patient, not because of his own needs for acceptance. Given its energizing effect, this caring is in itself a form of self-care.

The nurse narrative that follows illustrates the features of self-care that are foundational for effective adaptation to nursing practice. The story depicts Frances's experience of nursing school, her early enthusiasm for nursing, her growing frustration and eventual rejection of the profession, and finally her thoughtful choice to return to nursing.

Frances's Story

As a child, Frances did not dream of becoming a nurse. Born in the mid-1940s, she assumed that she would go to college, get married, have children, and stay at home until the children were launched. She gave no thought to her life beyond the anticipated days as mother and homemaker. Her mother, aunts, and all her mother's friends had stayed at home to raise kids; this was what Frances also imagined.

The first 30 years of Frances's life pretty much followed the path of her early imagination. Shortly after she completed college in the mid-1960s, Frances married a smart, funny man who not only shared her love but was also handsome. In the space of four years she had two sons, and over the next decade her life unfolded much as she had pictured and without significant disruption. However, in her thirties, with both children in school, Frances began to feel restless and to consider midlife career options. One day as she flipped through a catalogue of the programs of study at the local university, Frances noted the curriculum for the school of nursing. She recalled the spontaneity of her decision. "I'll be a nurse," she thought. "They take care of people, and I enjoy that. In fact, I'm pretty good at caring for my family. I could finish the degree in about three years and I like science. Yes, I'll become a nurse." When the next semester opened, with the full support of her husband and children, Frances began working toward her BSN degree.

She recalled those early student days: "I was a good student and I loved the challenge, but I was totally overwhelmed by the work. For two semesters I had classes on two days for six hours straight without a significant break. There were skills labs to attend, papers to write, clinical preparation, reading up to 400 pages a week for my classes, and studying for tests. It was incredibly stressful. For three years I juggled my schoolwork and family responsibilities. There was never time for myself, for a quiet cup of coffee or lunch with a friend. The time pressures were unbelievable, and the work was both emotionally and physically challenging. I had never been around sick people or seen a dead person, much less been with someone who was dying. Adding to the stress, the whole experience was permeated with the threat that everything I was supposed to learn was important and could either save a patient's life or kill the patient. Faculty would tell us, 'This is really important. Be sure you learn this.' But there was no way I could learn everything."

However, Frances thrived on challenges. She reflected, "Because nursing school seemed a worthwhile challenge and I was not a quitter, I was motivated to stick with it and to excel. I did not have any idea what I was getting into when I chose to become a nurse."

Frances's graduation from nursing school was tainted by her realization that the relationship with her husband had deteriorated. They were divorced shortly after she began her first nursing job on a medical-surgical unit. Heartbroken, Frances immersed herself in her work, focusing on mastering the skills she had practiced as a student. She took pride in her nursing and felt great satisfaction when she had time to actually care for patients as she had been taught in nursing school. Recalling her early nursing career, Frances said, "I was pretty overwhelmed with all the things I had to learn, but I loved it. I focused on learning new procedures, becoming familiar with new drugs, and developing my assessment skills. Sometimes I felt like a detective trying to find the clue that would lead to the best way to help a patient. While the work was harder than I had expected, I felt good mastering skills and working with patients."

Frances described a particularly meaningful afternoon about six months after her graduation. "I was caring for five patients, one of whom was dying. I had never had sole responsibility for a dying patient before, and I was both expectant and scared. Recalling what I had learned about care for the dying, I set about to meet the needs of the patient and the family. I remember recognizing that there was really nothing to 'do' for the patient but to keep him clean, dry, and free from pain. He was largely unconscious. His family, however, needed lots of reassurance, which as a new nurse, I gave by repeatedly taking his blood pressure and reporting the results to them. This seemed to comfort both of us. At one point they asked me if I could stay in the patient's room with them for a while. I remember my surprise at realizing that, in their eyes, I was a real nurse who knew what I was doing! I spent as much time as I could with the family and was at the patient's bedside when he died. In retrospect it is almost amusing—I was not sure he had died because his breathing had been so irregular. However, eventually I took his blood pressure and then I knew he was dead. I know that sounds crazy, but I was very inexperienced in these matters. I told the family, 'He is gone,' and we wept together. That experience was a critical one in my career. It highlighted what I loved about nursing. I had been welcomed into the private and sacred experience of the death of a beloved husband and father whom I did not even really know. I was ecstatic for several days."

Frances found, however, that moments of poignant human connection became harder and harder for her to experience. About a year after her graduation, she arrived at work on an evening shift to learn than two colleagues had called in sick and there was no one to replace them. Frances's workload was doubled. With the help of an LPN, she was responsible for 12 patients. The LPN was a capable nurse but legally was not allowed to give IV medications. Five of the patients were postop and were receiving IV antibiotics and IV pain management. To make matters worse, the division clerk who transcribed physician orders left midshift with a migraine headache, leaving Frances responsible for transcribing orders for all 12 of the patients. Her colleagues were equally overworked and could not help her. Frances explained, "The evening was impossible. There was no way I could provide safe care for all these patients. That night two incident reports were filed on me because I was late hanging IV antibiotics for two patients. To make matters worse, one of my patients was a sweet, quiet man who was dying. I could not spend much time with him. He wanted to talk, but I was rushing in and out of his room like a crazy person. It was just awful to have to turn away from his needs, but there was no time."

This shift marked the point when Frances faced the disparity between the ideal of nursing that she had been taught in nursing school and the reality of nursing. She became discouraged and angry. She felt increasingly unappreciated by management and frustrated when she could not practice nursing the way she felt it should be practiced. Frances recalled, "I began to realize that what mattered to me as a nurse, like spending time with the dying man on that frantic evening shift, was not a priority for the organization. No one wrote an incident report on me for not spending time with a dying patient. The organization only cared whether I hung my IV meds on time. I know that is important, but it is also important to comfort a dying patient. I had been trying to be an ideal nurse with every patient, and there was no way to do that and no energy or time left for me. So I began to shut down to everything at work after that shift; I felt trapped. It occurred to me to talk to my superiors, but everybody else was complaining and it did no good. I didn't want to be seen as a whiner. So I just showed up and did my job. I was determined no one was going to write another incident report on me."

Over the next two years, Frances grew increasingly dissatisfied with nursing. She recalled, "I focused on all the negatives. I couldn't see the positive aspects of my work. I felt that the nurse manager was unresponsive to my needs. I began to see patients as mostly demanding, and I grew increasingly disgruntled. Finally I quit. I wasn't even sad about quitting. I was just relieved. I still wanted to help others, but I decided nursing was not for me."

Frances began a new job as volunteer coordinator for the local hospice. At first she felt great relief. She no longer had to deal with her frustration over unmet patient needs and a system that did not seem to value her skills. There were disgruntled coworkers in her new job and managers who were not always responsive, but at least the pressure of taking care of sick people was gone. Frances smiled as she said, "Yet believe it or not, it didn't take long for me to begin to miss those sick people."

About eight months into her new job, Frances was conducting a volunteer hospice training session when a question by a volunteer led her to reflect on her decision to leave nursing. She recounted, "I was explaining to the volunteers how their work included listening to family fears and concerns about the dying patient when a young woman asked, 'What's it like to be with someone when they die?' Her question provoked a flood of memories from my nursing experience. I began to tell the volunteers about Don, Lawrence, Anita, and others for whom I had cared. Brave Don, who when he died said, 'I put up a damn good fight. Now I am very tired.' Lawrence, a father and grandfather, who several hours before he died, spoke for the first time in several days to reassure his family, 'You will be OK. I must go now.' Anita, a young mother whose wishes to be alert for her husband and child kept her from taking morphine until close to the end, when she said to me, 'I'll take that morphine now, and I thank you for your goodness to me.' As I recounted these stories, I was deeply touched by my memories of these patients. As I caught a glimpse of myself caring for them, I began to recognize that caring was my calling and I was good at it."

Over the next months, Frances realized that in her short nursing career her life had intersected with many individuals in deeply personal ways. Her reflections highlighted for her the richness and value of her work. Her musings were further stimulated by a call from her sister, who worked in the business world. Excited, Frances's sister reported that she had gone to a nursing home in her community to play hymns for the residents. "It was so satisfying. I felt like I was actually helping people," her sister exclaimed. Frances remembered thinking: "Nurses help people all the time. What other profession affords these opportunities?"

Over the next months, Frances continued to think about her patients. She also went to see a counselor to help her clarify options. After much thought, she decided to return to nursing. She enrolled in nursing school for her master's degree with the goal of working as an adult nurse practitioner (ANP) with a focus in oncology. Much had changed in the practice arena. Managed care had made its mark upon nursing and hospital patients were sicker. Frances reflected, "The system had changed but so had I. What was different for me was that this time around I knew what I was getting into and I still wanted to be a nurse. I wanted to be a nurse because, despite the hard work, I wanted to be a part of the experiences of my patients. I don't think I needed to leave nursing in the first place. If I had sought guidance, someone could have helped me see that I had options beyond feeling frustrated and victimized and I could have figured this out without leaving."

Frances completed her graduate studies and returned to work. Her attitude and approach to her work had changed, and she had chosen to work in oncology, a nursing specialty that allowed her to capitalize on her strengths and the values of caring and compassion. "I chose to go back into nursing in an area where I knew I could best use my skills," she explained. "I love helping patients deal with the symptoms of their disease and understand about chemotherapy. I love managing medications to keep patients comfortable, helping patients, and most of all, I love supporting patients through the experience of cancer from diagnosis to discharge or death."

Frances was now working in a specialty that she loved. The work was still demanding and every day was not a good one for Frances. Sometimes she felt that she did not have anything to give her patients. At times she felt weighed down by sadness for herself and for patients. Her work was especially hard when her personal life was troubled. She recalled an occasion when a long-term relationship with a boyfriend ended at the same time she was taking care of a young man with Hodgkin's disease. Her patient was bright, beautiful, and not doing well. "I remember him well, wearing a red baseball cap to conceal his baldness. He was a philosopher-type and he used to talk about the meaning of life and of his illness. One day he declared, 'No matter what cap I wear, I'm still a bald man in a hat.' Another time he observed, 'I've never been in love, what is that like?' I remember thinking that there wasn't any goodness in this. I had to look closely to see that the gift for me was witnessing his courage and beauty. For him, I don't know what the goodness could have been. Perhaps my care and attentiveness offered a small comfort. The day he died I was deeply sad. It was almost too much for me. My boyfriend was gone and I remember thinking, 'I can't cope without some support.' So I went to some of my nurse colleagues and fell into their arms and sobbed. They were good nurses, so they knew what to do—they didn't say a word, they just held me while I sobbed, 'Life is so unfair. He was so good and young and beautiful.' I think I was crying for both of us because life isn't fair. Nursing teaches hard lessons."

As Frances's expertise developed, she recognized the need for some respite from the daily challenges of cancer patients. So she negotiated an expansion of her role. She wrote a teaching module for patients undergoing chemotherapy. She started a bereavement group for family members. She began to meet with staff nurses to help problem solve pain-related concerns of oncology patients. Branching out in her work, she contributed to the needs of the organization while creating variety for herself. Frances explained, "My work in oncology has its own strains and grief—from the diagnosis of cancer, the trauma of treatment and the transition to recovery or death. I had to take approaches to my work that were less stressful. My projects worked for me and the organization."

Reflecting on her role, Frances said, "I love my work. I also have days when I would rather stay at home. But that would be true for any job. I stay in nursing because the potential is always there for a rich human connection, even when I am most weary and needing a break. Positive encounters with patients energize me. Let me tell you one more story to show you what I mean," she added.

"Last week I was running out of steam. I needed a day off, and because of staffing problems, I could not get it. I went by to check on a patient who had begun radiation treatments that morning for cancer of the anus. He was shy, pretty unsophisticated, and ill at ease in the hospital setting. He was from a rural area and had never traveled or been away from his family before. He was alone that day. When I went in to his room, he was sitting on the bed in bright new yellow pajamas, the top still creased in the front. He was so upset he was wringing his hands. It seemed no one had told him the details of his radiation therapy. He had not realized he would have to position himself under the machine with his backside up in the air, exposed to the young female nurse. He was mortified. I listened as he talked of his humiliation and recognized my connection to him as he lamented, 'You know, it's about man's inhumanity to man.'

'Yes, I do know,' I replied. We shared this understanding and this created a tie between us that reminded me of why I am a nurse. My role is to humanize the inhumanity of treatments, protocols, technology and the system itself with my care and compassion. That is the joy of my work. It helps the patient and it keeps me human."

Frances has now been working as an ANP in oncology for four years. She describes the work as "wonderful and terrible" at the same time. "Opposites abound in the work," she says. "Without the human misery there would be no need for compassion. Without the organization and all its weaknesses, there would be no framework for my work. Without the suffering there would be no joy. Without the feelings of being overwhelmed, I could not feel the satisfaction of mastery of my work. Without my wonderful patients, I wouldn't have all these great stories to tell. The important thing for me is to engage in the struggle of these opposites. When I no longer struggle with opposites, including my own need to relieve patient suffering and my inability at times to do so, then I will be numb. For now, nursing works well for me. If I become numb to the human feelings and experiences around me, I hope I'll have enough wisdom to leave."

Enacting Artful Nursing

Caring for oneself in a profession like nursing requires vigilance and perseverance. Frances left nursing because she felt unappreciated and could not consistently practice the ideals of the profession. Her return to nursing was motivated by a realization that caring encounters offer a joy and richness that are hard to replicate in other professions. Frances's return to nursing was marked by three features of caring for oneself:

- Making an informed choice
- Accepting responsibility
- Giving and receiving

MAKING AN INFORMED CHOICE

Frances's initial enthusiasm for her work was diminished by her feelings of burnout and her frustration at what she perceived to be her inability to practice the ideals of the profession. Focusing on the negative aspects of the role, Frances began to see herself as unappreciated and powerless and the patients as "mostly demanding." With a vision of herself as "trapped," Frances was in a poor position to take care of herself. Her story demonstrates the evolution of her choice to be a nurse from an initial naïve decision to enter nursing to an *informed* decision to return to nursing.

Obviously students of nursing have already made the choice to become a nurse. However, there is a catch-22 in that an *informed* choice to be a nurse is impossible without experience as a nurse. Like the development of nursing skills, the practice of nursing cannot be understood without experiencing it. While glimpses of what it means to be a nurse are available through exposure to nurses, without direct experience one cannot know what it means to practice nursing. Consider, for example, how your own views of nursing have changed between the time when you decided to become a nurse and now, when you have had some direct exposure to practice. Your choice to enter nursing may have been spontaneous, as it was for Frances, or thoughtful, prolonged, and even based on conversations or direct contact with nurses. However, until you have experience as a nurse, your choice cannot be fully informed.

Frances chose the profession because she had enjoyed caring for her own family and instinctively felt she would enjoy nursing. During the first three years of her practice, she began to recognize that she could not always practice the ideals of the profession and that nursing was hard work. Frances left nursing, unable to reconcile her ideals with the reality of the work. In so doing, she also turned away from what she soon came to recognize as the richness and value of nurses' work. Further, she realized that few professions other than nursing offer the rewards of caring for vulnerable persons. Having gained this knowledge, Frances returned to nursing. Her work was more demanding and the patients were sicker, yet Frances made a satisfactory and happy adjustment to her work. Recall her observation: "What was different for me [in terms of work satisfaction] was that I knew what I was getting into and I still wanted to be a nurse."

Frances was now in a position to take care of herself. Her focus had broadened to include a realistic appreciation of the whole of nursing. She had learned through experience that nursing involves ample occasions for feeling *either* proud or defeated, useful or used, affirmed or discounted, responsible or victimized, happy or disgruntled, satisfied or dissatisfied. She had felt all of these opposing feelings. She now took a proactive and positive approach as she set out to "humanize the inhumanity of treatments, protocols, technology, and the system itself with my care and compassion." This focus, Frances declared, "keeps me human." Contributing to her informed choice was Frances's careful assessment of her strengths and limitations. Recognizing that she thrived on caring connections with patients, she chose a specialty that offered ample opportunity for such encounters.

Informed choice is rarely easy because to be fully informed is to be aware of the full range of possibilities. It is not unusual for a patient to respond to the request to give an informed consent for a procedure with the statement, "Just do what you have to do. I don't want to know all the details. They upset me." Likewise, it is tempting as a new nurse to close one's eyes to "all the details" about what it means to be a nurse. However, until one is willing to see the full range of challenges and joys in nursing, as well as one's own strengths and limitations, there is no informed consent. Without informed choice, there is little possibility for self-care—only victimization, frustration and burnout.

ACCEPTING RESPONSIBILITY

Initially, Frances's response to the organization's indifference to her needs was to feel helpless. She recalled feeling, "There was nothing I could do." She did not even try to talk to those in charge of her unit, since "everybody was complaining and it did no good. I didn't want to be seen as a whiner." Choosing to see herself as a victim rather than risk being seen as a complainer, Frances remained stuck in her helplessness and frustration. She took no responsibility for improving her work situation; she simply blamed others. In short order, Frances became so dissatisfied she quit nursing without any feelings of sadness about leaving a profession she had once loved.

In order to return to nursing with success and satisfaction, Frances had to accept personal responsibility for all that was entailed in her choice to be a nurse. She could no longer claim the innocence and blamelessness of a victim. Rather than succumb to burnout after her return to nursing, Frances became proactive, working creatively to expand her role. Instead of leaving a system that did not entirely support the ideals of nursing, she set out to humanize the dehumanizing aspects of the system; system challenges became opportunities to practice the ideals of nursing within an imperfect organization.

No longer expecting the work setting to be consistently supportive or to reward her for caring, Frances took responsibility for maintaining her commitment to caring while getting her own needs met. Support came from her joy in working with patients. For example, unable to see any goodness in her young patient's dying, she found the hidden gift of his courage and beauty. Horrified by the humiliation of the man with cancer of the anus, she reached out to comfort him, comforting herself as well with the reminder of their shared humanity. At times Frances sought the support of colleagues. Grieving over her patient's death and her own personal loss, she turned to other nurses who held her as she sobbed.

Taking personal responsibility for one's choice to be a nurse enables one to also take responsibility for self-care. Personal responsibility is vital if the nurse is to flourish in the professional role.

GIVING AND RECEIVING

In an account of caring for her son Max, born with multiple physical problems, a mother declared, "The truth is that Max has made me more deeply happy than I have ever been. . . . He changes everyone who meets him. He changes their ideas about beauty, about worth. He has made every member of our family—immediate as well as extended—grow up and change their life view in some essential way" (Franks, 1999, p. 77). Most of us have a deep longing to give to others, to have meaningful work, and to experience love. Indeed, some claim that it is a form of human suffering not to find a way to give of oneself (Brussat & Brussat, 1996).

Despite the deep human impulse to care, it is not easy to do so day after day in one's work. Central to success is learning how to receive from others, especially patients. At first it may sound contradictory to speak of the nurse *receiving* from the patient. The chapter on caring noted that the focus of the nurse is on the patient and the patient's needs, rather than the needs of the nurse. However, each story in this text testifies to the richness of caring encounters for the nurse. Reciprocity of caring, whereby the one caring *and* the one cared for benefit from the caring encounter, has long been recognized as key to nurse satisfaction (Vezeau, 1992).

Reciprocity in caring occurs when the nurse is open to the patient's reality "as a possibility for my own" (Noddings, 1984, p. 14). With this appreciation, the nurse is deeply touched by the plight of the other, aware that "this could be me, or someone I love." Acting to "eliminate the intolerable, to reduce the pain, to fill the need, to actualize the dream" (Noddings, p. 14), the one caring "receive[s] the other into myself, and I see and feel with the other. I become a duality . . . I feel what he says he felt. I have been invaded by the other . . . [and] I shall never again be completely without regard for him" (pp. 30–31).

Each nurse-patient encounter is different; hence the nurse receives the patient expectantly, recognizing that every encounter contains possibilities for human connection and "a lifetime burning in every moment" (Eliot, 1963, p. 189). Every nurse-patient encounter holds the promise of a deeply satisfying experience, but in reality, not all encounters are ideal. However, on those occasions when the nurse and patient are connected at a deeply human level, both are enriched. Thus, caring holds the possibility of self-care in the form of personal satisfaction. Indeed, given the rewards of giving and receiving, when the nurse cares for others, he is also caring for himself. Recognizing this certainty, Frances learned that she alone could not change the health care system, but she could ameliorate patient loneliness and suffering by "humanizing the inhumanity" of health care delivery, all the while enriching and changing her own reality.

Challenges to Caring for Oneself

This chapter opened with a discussion of three major factors that challenge self-care: burnout, professional dynamics, and personal responses to nursing. While these affect all nurses, they represent only the beginning in terms of work-related challenges to caring for oneself. The challenges are legion. How can the new nurse best care for herself in the face of the multiple demands of the work setting?

Self-care requires paying attention to environmental challenges that may be depleting—for instance, colleagues who are unpleasant and uncooperative; a physical work environment that is crowded or noisy; or multiple patients whose needs are excessive or whose personal style is demanding, angry, or uncooperative. Whatever the depleting situation, it is important to see it for what it is. Without recognition, the situation chips away at the nurse's well-being.

Once the offending situation is recognized, the nurse needs to decide what can be changed, what is likely not to change, and what are the options. For example, if your patient workload has been extremely challenging for an extended period of time, you could try to take time away from patients. Perhaps you could update nurse protocols, work at the desk, take a day off, or even arrange to work in a less demanding unit for a few weeks (Burr, 1996; Kennedy & Barloon, 1997). Creative problem solving is key to self-care (Kennedy & Barloon, 1997). What is most important, however, is not so much *what* you do but that you *do something* to confront what is becoming intolerable (Burr, 1996). Taking action is key. If you act on your behalf, you will not feel like a victim. By avoiding a victim stance, you are in a position to take care of yourself.

Some challenges to self-care, such as poor management or unrelenting heavy workloads, are beyond the power of the individual nurse to change.

When one is faced with an "unworkable" situation, one must make a choice informed by the realities of the situation, one's own strengths and limitations, and the viable options. The role of informed choice cannot be overstated. Work stress is reduced by assuming responsibility for choosing the type of work one does and knowing the reasons for that choice (Burr, 1996). The effects of informed choice on Frances's work satisfaction and self-care were indisputable.

It is also helpful to recognize the dynamic nature of nursing and your own growth as a nurse. You will grow in fits and starts, and your career may take many forms. Thus self-care includes an ongoing assessment of your vision of your career, the influences on your career decisions, and your career itself (Hobbs, 1998).

You will grow in fits and starts, and the work environment will always be in a state of flux and change. Self-care involves paying attention to changes in nursing and making them work for you rather than seeing them as threats (Vicenzi, White, & Begun, 1997). Successful adaptation to inevitable changes in nursing entails abandoning the hope of always controlling work-related changes, accepting the reality that change is inevitable, tolerating the unpredictability of the future, building relationships with colleagues, and "taking responsibility for lifelong learning to keep your skills fresh and to build new ones" (Vicenzi et al., 1997, p. 28).

One key to self-care is self-knowledge (Hobbs, 1998). Self-knowledge illuminates your needs and helps you recognize when to say no to extra demands. Self-knowledge also helps you engage in honest reflections about the reasons you became a nurse; envision your own dreams as a nurse; realistically assess your motivations and limitations, and the strengths you bring to your career; and honestly appraise alternatives and opportunities when faced with career-related challenges (Hobbs, 1998). Nurses who are realistic about work and expect to encounter a reasonable number of work-related problems are less likely to suffer burnout than those who fail to acknowledge work-related difficulties (Duquette et al., 1994). Further, acknowledgment of work-related challenges leads to creative problem solving (Kennedy & Barloon, 1997). Finally, self-knowledge involves noting early signs of burnout and knowing when to seek help from mentors or counselors (Burr, 1996).

It is not easy to take care of yourself in nursing. It may be even more difficult to take care of yourself as a student of nursing. Occasionally faculty or preceptors exert power *over* a student rather than engaging *with* the student in problem solving or learning (Roberts, 1998). This kind of oppression is not always intentional; it may result from a teaching or precepting style that involves telling students what to do rather than empowering students to problem solve with help (Roberts, 1998).

Most students have felt disempowered at some point by faculty or preceptors. As difficult as these occasions are, they present an opportunity for you to begin to develop skills in self-care. Recognizing the challenging situation is the first step; the next is assessing one's options realistically. Can the preceptor or faculty member be approached directly for a dialogue about the situation? Is there someone you can turn to for support or help in problem solving? Is the situation one you simply have to tolerate until the experience ends? Regardless of the outcome of the situation, the actions of noticing, assessing, and problem solving offer occasions for moving away from the role of victim and honing self-care skills that will serve you well in your nursing career.

Summary

Caring for oneself is not an option if the nurse is to thrive and grow in the nursing role. There are multiple obstacles to self-care, including feelings of burnout and professional and personal dynamics that promote excessive self-sacrifice. Key to self-care is making an informed choice to be a nurse and accepting responsibility for that choice. In so doing, the nurse avoids feelings of victimization that lead to anger and burnout. Vigilance in regard to internal and external factors that inhibit self-care and a receptive attitude to reciprocity between nurse and patient set the stage for self-care in nursing.

References

Beck, C.T. (1995). Burnout in undergraduate nursing students. *Nurse Educator, 20*(4), 19–23.

Brussat, F., & Brussat, M.A. (1996). *Spiritual literacy.* New York: Simon and Schuster.

Burr, C.K. (1996). Supporting the helpers. *Nursing Clinics of North America, 31*, 243–251.

Caffey, R.A., & Caffey, P.A. (1994). Nursing: Caring or codependent? *Nursing Forum, 29*(1), 12–17.

Duquette, A., Kerouac, S., Sandhu, B.K., & Beaudet, L. (1994). Factors related to nursing burnout: A review of empirical knowledge. *Issues in Mental Health Nursing, 15*, 337–358.

Eliot, T.S. (1963). *Collected poems 1909–1962.* New York: Harcourt, Brace and Company.

Farrington, A. (1997). Strategies for reducing stress and burnout in nursing. *British Journal of Nursing, 6*, 44–50.

Franks, L. (1999). Miracle kid. *The New Yorker,* May, pp. 68–77.

Freire, P. (1971). *Pedagogy of the oppressed.* New York: Herder & Herder.

Haack, M. (1988). Stress and impairment among nursing students. *Research in Nursing Health, 11,* 125–134.

Hobbs, B.B. (1998). Taking charge of your career. *American Journal of Nursing, 98,* 36–40.

Keen, P. (1991). Caring for ourselves. In R.M. Neil & R. Watts (Eds.), *Caring and nursing: Explorations in feminist perspectives* (pp. 173–187). New York: National League for Nursing.

Kennedy, D., & Barloon, L.F. (1997). Managing burnout in pediatric critical care: The human care commitment. *Critical Care Nursing Quarterly, 20*(2), 63–71.

Kushnir, R., Rabin, S., & Azulai, S. (1997). A descriptive study of stress management in a group of pediatric oncology nurses. *Cancer Nursing, 20,* 414–419.

McCall, E. (1996). Horizontal violence in nursing: The continued silence. *Lamp, 53*(3), 28–29, 31.

Molassiotis, A., & Haberman, M. (1996). Evaluation of burnout and job satisfaction in marrow transplant nurses. *Cancer Nursing, 19,* 360–367.

Noddings, N. (1984). *Caring: A feminine approach to ethics & moral education.* Berkeley: University of California Press.

Pike, A.W. (1997). Engaging collegial relationships: The demise of nurse as victim. In J.C. McCloskey & H.K. Grace (Eds.), *Current issues in nursing* (pp. 532–536). St. Louis: Mosby.

Reverby, S. (1987). *Ordered to care: The dilemma of American nursing.* New York: Cambridge University Press.

Roberts, S.J. (1983). Oppressed group behavior: Implications for nursing. *Advances in Nursing Science,* July, 21–30.

Roberts, S.J. (1998). Health promotion as empowerment: Suggestions for changing the balance of power. *Clinical Excellence for Nurse Practitioners, 2,* 183–187.

Swartzky, J. (1996). Stress in critical care nurses: Actual and perceived. *Heart and Lung, 25,* 409–417.

Vezeau, T.M. (1992). Caring: From philosophical concerns to practice. *The Journal of Clinical Ethics, 3,* 18–20.

Vicenzi, A.E., White, K.R., & Begun, J.W. (1997). Chaos in nursing: Make it work for you. *American Journal of Nursing, 97*(10), 26–31.

Warner, C.G., Black, V.L., & Parent, P.C. (1998). Image of nursing. In G. Deloughery (Ed.), *Issues and trends in nursing* (pp. 390–409). St. Louis: Mosby.

APPLICATION

....

ACTIVITY I
Group Discussion: Analysis of the Story

1. What do you think about the way Frances made her decision to become a nurse? Some believe that the best nurses are "called" to be a nurse. What are your thoughts about that claim?

2. What would you have done differently from Frances when she was caring for her first dying patient? Explain your reasons.

3. Recall the extremely difficult shift after which Frances began to face the disparity between the ideal of nursing as she had been taught in nursing school and the reality of nursing. At this point she began to "just show up" and do her job. What other options could Frances have chosen?

4. After Frances returned to nursing, she began to take better care of herself while at work. Discuss the ways she cared for herself in her work. Can you think of other things she might have done that would have helped sustain her in her work?

ACTIVITY II
Group Discussion: Confronting Reality

1. Discuss any differences you can identify between the ideal nurse as depicted in your classes in nursing school and the nurses you have seen in practice.

2. Discuss factors that influence self-care that might explain these differences?

3. Describe any differences between what you have been taught as the ideal of nursing practice and what you have found to be true in your clinical experiences.

4. How do you explain these differences?

ACTIVITY III
Group Discussion: Why I Want To Be a Nurse

1. Say why you made the choice to be a nurse. Include in your statement any specific event that influenced your choice.

2. Describe what you have learned about nursing that most disappoints you. State how you plan to deal with this disappointment.

3. Describe what it is about nursing that most interests you. State how you hope to capitalize on this feature of nursing.

ACTIVITY IV
Self-Reflection: Confronting Challenges

Complete the following statements:

1. In regard to burnout and my practice as a nurse, I am most concerned about

2. The strengths that I bring to this concern include

3. Things I can do to increase my skills in dealing with this concern include

4. The thing that makes it hard for me to say no when someone asks me to take on extra work is

5. Identify two occasions when you said yes when someone asked you to do something and you did not want to do it.

Examine your motives on these two occasions. Why did you say yes?

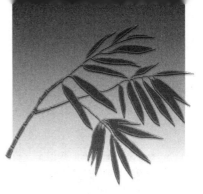

Index